Dedication

THIS BOOK is dedicated to James Eyer; Louis R. Caplan, MD; Daniel C. Randa, MD; and Professor Joseph Maiolo, four friends who believed in me and helped me to develop once impossible dreams into today's realities.

IN MEMORY OF
David K. Nelson

After a Stroke

300
Tips for Making Life Easier

by Cleo Hutton

Demos

Demos Medical Publishing
386 Park Avenue South
New York, NY 10016, USA

Designed and produced by Reyman Studio

Visit our website at www.demosmedpub.com
http://www.demosmedicalpub.com

Library of Congress Cataloging-in-Publication Data

    Hutton, Cleo, 1949-
    After a stroke : 300 tips to making life easier / by Cleo Hutton.
    p. cm.
Includes index.
ISBN 1-932603-11-5 (pbk. : alk. paper)
1. Cerebrovascular disease—Popular works. I. Title.
RC388.5.H879 2005
616.8'103—dc22

                               2005007542

Photos courtesy of North Coast Medical, Inc
18305 Sutter Boulevard
Morgan Hill, CA 95037-2845
www.ncmedical.com
www.BeAbleToDo.com

Printed in Canada

Acknowledgments

THANK YOU to Diana M. Schneider, PhD, President and Publisher at Demos Medical Publishing, Inc., Ruth Toda, Managing Editor, Sharon S. Ballas and Joann Woy for their assistance with editing and publishing After a Stroke: 300 Tips for Making Life Easier. We hope you, the reader, find the tips useful on your journey toward recovery.

Thank you to Roy Beckham, Director of Marketing Communications and Jeri Francis, Graphics Designer at North Coast Medical, Inc., for the use of images from the North Coast Medical, Inc. Functional Solutions catalogue.

Contents

Section VII – Brain Builders

Section VIII –
The Importance of Love

Preface

A STROKE STRUCK YOU or someone you love. You have gone through the critical stage of this devastating condition and perhaps even graduated from a hospital rehabilitation program. Now, you begin another phase of rehabilitation, as your battle for recovery is showing undeniable progress: You're going home. The purpose of this book is to give you helpful tips and information about stroke that will serve as necessary artillery to help you overcome obstacles in the way of successful healing at home.

I am your peer, a fellow stroke survivor/hero who has experienced some of the emotions and physical limitations you may be feeling today. My new career is that of an author and speaker on the topic of stroke awareness and recovery from a personal perspective. This is an unexpected achievement. Twelve years ago, I could not write, speak, walk, organize thought processes, see using the left visual field, remember or interpret directions or language, or move my affected left side. It is, quite simply, wonderful to have progressed so far. Despite two devastating strokes, I remained focused on rehabilitation, medical information, training, education, stroke issues, adaptability, creativity, and stroke-related resources. I am simply a facilitator, gathering facts and experience and relating to others what I have learned about rehabilitation and stroke issues.

Stroke awareness is the cornerstone of stroke prevention. I have great respect and admiration for our brain power. Mainly, this reverence comes from experiencing many of the devastating effects of stroke and the long process involved in recovery. Also, the nursing skills I acquired before my stroke continue to assist me in understanding medical terminology related to stroke care. *After a Stroke: 300 Tips for Making Life Easier* will give you, the reader, creative tips I have learned along a 12-year course of continuous rehabilitation through everyday living.

Before giving tips, it is important to review general information about stroke so that we can use this, too, as a tool in our recovery process. This book is not intended to replace, or infringe upon, your physician's medical advice. I am not a doctor. Your physician and medical team have the expertise and training necessary to attend to your medical care.

The brain is complex. Stroke affects every individual differently. This diversity is caused by the location of the obstructed artery supplying blood to locations within the brain, the extent of permanently injured brain areas, and the type of stroke: hemorrhagic or ischemic.

A *hemorrhagic stroke* occurs when a blood vessel bursts within the brain, causing blood to spill into spaces surrounding brain cells. This type of stroke can happen because of several reasons. A head injury is one example. Another reason may be an *aneurysm*, a bulging blood vessel wall within the brain. Usually, an aneurysm is treated surgically. This is the most dangerous form of stroke.

Ischemic stroke is the most common type. It is caused by a blockage of blood flow to areas within the brain. This kind of stroke may happen because of an *embolism*, a blood clot that originates from anywhere in the body and is sent through the circulatory system, to eventually clog a small blood vessel and prevent blood from circulating. An analogy is to think of a stream of water supplying a fertile valley with nutrients that help flowers grow, crops flourish, and grasslands develop. Now, imagine large stones or boulders falling into the stream, creating a dam so that no water reaches the valley. Soon, without the water supply, the valley dries up, nothing grows, and the vegetation dies. That is what an embolism (boulder) causes within a blood vessel (stream) of the brain (fertile valley). When a specific part of the brain is deprived of blood flow, that brain area no longer functions, and it dies. In turn, the body function regulated by that particular brain area is affected.

The left side of your brain controls the right side of your body and vice versa. *Hemiplegia* means that a person has paralysis or weakness on one side of the body. The standard medical explanation for stroke deficits is that if a stroke occurs in the right side of the brain, a person may have hemiplegia of the left-sided body, vision difficulties, sudden curious behavior, and loss of memory. If stroke affects the left side of the brain, a person may have right-sided hemiplegia, language and speech difficulties, and slow cautious behavior, along with memory loss. However, if stroke affects several brain areas because a blood clot breaks up and clogs various brain centers, however, this standard may not apply, and the problem becomes more complex. All too often, the medical community and others compartmentalize people who have a stroke into a strictly right or left brain stroke, depending on their affected side or hemiplegia. However, the stroke may have affected other brain areas as well. Your neurologist and medical team will be able to give you the best advice about the stroke you had and what body functions are affected.

* It is extremely important to have your neurologist explain to you and your family the exact brain areas, and their functions, affected by your particular stroke.

Another analogy that further explains how stroke affects the brain is to think of the brain as the world. Airports have airplanes that take off and land every second throughout the entire world, just as our brain has major centers that allow our body to function. The airlines at these cerebral airports are called *neurons*. These neurons send electrical impulses—we'll call them passengers—traveling from one point to another within our global brain, carrying with them patterns that form our personality, behavior, and emotions. These passengers also tell our body to see, hear, remember, reason, problem solve, feel, and automatically instruct our heart to beat and lungs to breathe, among other duties. These little neurons/airlines and impulses/passengers are busy even when we are sleeping. When a blood clot occurs within our brain-world, a major airport may shut down for a short time, as in a *transient ischemic attack (TIA)*, or permanently, as in a stroke. The impulses/passengers can no longer get to their destinations. Sometimes, the neurons begin to erratically send off impulses in wrong directions, causing an overload of electrical impulses or *seizures*. When an airport or airports closes permanently, as in a stroke, the passengers who traveled through that airport are also affected. If you can't move an arm or leg, it is because the neurons/airlines communicating to the major brain center/airport in controlling that particular movement is closed. Just as a closed airport is not routing passengers to their proper destinations, neither are neurons carrying message impulses to move your arm or leg. For example, if the neurons at the hippocampus airport in our brain are closed down, it will affect our ability to learn and remember. If the frontal cortex region is affected, our emotions, reasoning, and thinking skills go awry because the impulses don't arrive at their proper destinations. Other brain centers have additional important duties in routing their particular impulses. Depression can be a devastating side effect of stroke when neurons transmitting emotional wellness, happiness, or comfort are affected. Medications may be needed to blunt the number of erratic electrical impulses from flooding our brain-world.

How can we ever recover from stroke when brain areas are effectively shut down and impulses are whizzing in wrong directions? Like an airport faced with a disaster, our brain is as adaptable and creative as people in our outside world are when tragedy strikes. In the brain, this is called *plasticity*. Depending on the neuron and brain center affected, other brain centers can be trained to reroute impulses to use different neurons. After a stroke, the brain-world will forever remain altered, just as the airport (or portion of the airport, depending on the extent of the upheaval) cannot function as before. Therapy teaches the neurons to use alternative routes to guide electrical impulses. *Constraint-induced therapy* restrains the unaffected side of our body to force neurons into transmitting messages through alternative routes around the stroke-affected brain areas. As in any form of learning, these patterns must be repeated until the brain centers and neurons become skilled at developing alternative routes for their impulses through undamaged neurons, thus minimizing the loss of body functions. This tremendously efficient and adaptable brain-world controls all body functions and contains everything concerning who we are.

In 1992, when I had a stroke, stroke patient care was handled differently. *Tissue plasminogen activator (TPA)*, a clot-dissolving drug sometimes given within the first 3 hours of the onset of ischemic stroke to combat further damage, was not available at the community hospital I was admitted to. Today, many hospitals have *Stroke Centers* that specialize in immediate stroke care. These hospital centers make a great difference in promptly diagnosing and treating stroke patients. But at that time, as my brain swelled from progressively damaged areas, the neurologist followed a "wait and see" protocol. As I slept, more brain areas became ischemic and died due to lack of blood flow. Luckily, a cardiologist diagnosed that the strokes had originated from a *congenital heart condition* (a heart defect that I was born with), and heart surgery avoided further episodes. But, by then, damage from multiple ischemic strokes was evident. Seizures developed over the following 2 years. After intense in- and outpatient rehabilitation, it was finally time for me to recover at home. I struggled with the feeling of being abandoned by helpful therapists and wondered how to manage various day-to-day problems and tasks. At first, I did not realize that I was using creative techniques to problem-solve, thereby encouraging new connections within my brain. I just wanted to get better. After going through, coming back, and going through again, all the emotional phases of adjustment associated with stroke and this traumatic life-changing event, I decided to use time to my advantage. Along with prescribed medications, I took a healthy dose of optimism. In the following chapters, you will discover tips that can aid in your emotional recovery, too.

Other medical conditions may slow down your progress in stroke recovery. Some situations include risk factors that contributed to stroke, such as heart disease, high blood pressure (also called *hypertension*), high LDL cholesterol levels, and diabetes mellitus. However, hypertension, elevated *LDL* (low-density lipoprotein; bad cholesterol) or low levels of *HDL* (high-density lipoprotein; good cholesterol), or diabetes can be controlled by medication and diet. Heart disease is closely related to stroke. Therefore, heart conditions mandate close supervision by a *cardiologist*, a physician specializing in the practice of *cardiovascular* (heart function) medicine.

The heart pumps blood rich in oxygen and other nutrients necessary for our brain to function. *Atrial fibrillation*, a rhythm disorder within the upper chambers of the heart, or *carotid artery disease*, a narrowing of one or both carotid arteries on each side of the neck caused by the build-up of fatty deposits called *atherosclerosis*, are high risk factors for stroke. A blood clot or particle of fat that is routed to our brain from anywhere in our arterial *circulatory system* (heart, blood vessels, and arteries) can cause a stroke.

Peripheral artery disease occurs when blood vessels in the leg or arm become narrowed with fatty deposits, and this condition can be a precursor to carotid artery disease and, possibly, stroke. An enlarged heart, heart valves that do not function properly, congenital heart defects, and of course heart disease, are factors in increasing your risk of stroke.

Some blood disorders carry a high risk of stroke too. *Sickle-cell anemia*, a genetic disorder mainly affecting African-Americans, causes the inability of red blood cells to carry oxygen and reduces the oxygen supply to organs. These malformed cells also tend to stick to blood vessel walls and may block the flow of blood to the brain, causing a stroke. Any blood disorder that causes a high red blood cell count has the potential to slow down the flow of blood to the point of forming clots. Physicians can treat this problem by monitoring your blood count through laboratory tests and prescribing medication that acts to speed up blood flow.

I am a Licensed Practical Nurse with several years of experience in the field of nursing. However, I did not see the warning signs of stroke when they were perfectly obvious in my life. I was young (43 years old at the time of the first major stroke) and naïve to circumstances that eventually changed my lifestyle. At times, I was unable to distinguish the severity of these symptoms because my brain was clouded by the marauding influence of stroke itself.

Transient ischemic attacks, also called *TIAs* or *mini-strokes*, are warning attacks that cause the same type of symptoms as stroke, but result in no significant loss of function. Recognizing and seeking immediate medical care if warning attacks occur can reduce your chances of having another stroke. These bothersome and mostly painless symptoms may last only a few minutes and disappear as quickly as they began. But TIAs could forecast that you are in danger of having a stroke. Here are the five warning signs of stroke defined by the American Heart Association/American Stroke Association and National Stroke Association. Seek immediate medical attention if you notice any of these warning signs:

1. Sudden numbness or weakness of the face, arm, or leg, especially on one side of the body
2. Sudden confusion, trouble speaking, or trouble understanding the written or spoken word
3. Sudden trouble seeing in one or both eyes
4. Sudden trouble walking, loss of balance, or coordination
5. Sudden severe headache with no known cause (hemorrhagic stroke)

Call 911. *Time equals brain.* This means that vital brain function is in jeopardy with every second the brain is without an adequate blood supply. It may be difficult for the person experiencing stroke warning signs to realize the severity of the symptoms. Remember, TIAs may affect a person's ability to think clearly or make reasonable choices. Everyone must be vigilant.

Obesity is another risk factor relating to stroke. This condition can lead to high blood pressure, diabetes, high cholesterol, and heart disease. *Obesity* is defined as an excess amount of body fat measured by using a mathematical formula based on a person's height and weight to reach *body mass index* or *BMI.* Obesity places a great strain on our heart and other systems within our bodies to keep working efficiently. The body may not be burning or consuming enough energy through exercise to adequately use the energy in food consumed. We can change our eating habits and make better choices of what types of foods we eat. This book will give you tips on dietary lifestyle options in the *Let's Get Cookin'* section, a new approach for your self-image in *Improving Self-Esteem,* as well as activities you may be able to accomplish after a stroke in *Let's Get Moving* and *Brain Builders.*

Also, it is important to understand that you cannot control some stroke risk factors. Here, our power is in knowledge gained. Many things in life are beyond our ability to change. Learning about them helps us deal with those issues. As we age, our risk factor for stroke increases. The incidence of stroke more than doubles each decade after age 55. Even our gender is a factor for stroke. Men have more strokes than women, but more women die of stroke than men. This could be because, on average, women live longer. If you have a family history of stroke, you also are at increased risk. African-Americans have a higher risk of death from stroke than Caucasians because they have higher incidences of high blood pressure and diabetes. These facts should keep us vigilant about our health issues while we learn to live again; we can rise above statistics and break paradigms regarding stroke.

Knowing your risk factors for stroke can significantly lessen your chance of another stroke occurring. Some risk factors we cannot change, such as our age, ethnic group, family history of coronary disease and/or stroke, sickle-cell anemia disease, and gender.

Now that you have had a stroke, the risk factor is increased for another incident unless the cause was found and alleviated. Even after finding the cause of your stroke, the risk may still be present, because your brain is weakened from the initial stroke. A 5-year stroke-free period post-stroke is usually used as an indicator that risk factors have been reduced.

Some risk factors we can change or medically treat to reduce our risk of stroke:

* Control high blood pressure, check it regularly, and see your physician for medical treatment.
* Diabetes mellitus can be controlled through medical intervention, diet, and insulin if required.
* Heart disease and/or atrial fibrillation can be medically treated, modified, or controlled through medication or surgery and frequent medical checkups.
* High LDL (bad cholesterol) or low levels of HDL (good cholesterol) can be treated through medications, diet, and exercise.

- Obesity can be lessened by diet and at least 30 minutes of vigorous cardiovascular exercise daily.
- Smoking or the use of any type of tobacco product must be halted, through medication or treatment.
- Alcohol abuse can be alleviated through treatment.
- Illegal drug use, such as cocaine use, must be immediately treated and stopped.
- Birth control pills or birth control patches carry a risk factor for stroke for women, especially if accompanied by smoking.
- Hormone replacement therapies carry the same risk factor for older women. Check with your physician about your particular risks.
- *Transient ischemic attacks* (TIAs) or mini-strokes are the forerunner or warning signs of stroke. Recognize the warning signs and immediately call for medical assistance if they occur. TIAs can be treated and can reduce your risk of having a major stroke.
- Sometimes the cost of an aspirin a day, a few cents, can alleviate a lifetime of stroke recovery and financial difficulties. However, do not take aspirin unless your physician has prescribed it for you, because aspirin may be an inadvisable treatment when taken with other medications.

The effects of stroke will change how you live. Hopefully, the modifications learned in therapy and continued at home with the aid of this book, will return you to an independent lifestyle. *After a Stroke: 300 Tips for Making Life Easier* will become a crucial part of your healing journey. My goal is to assist you as you develop longer periods of endurance, regain self-confidence, adjust to adaptabilities, create capabilities, call on courage, and increase your inner strength to achieve your fullest possible potential.

Rehabilitation began as soon as your neurologist determined that you were medically stable and could benefit from a somewhat rigorous routine of working toward recovery. Sometimes, rehabilitation began at your bedside while you were unable to attend formal therapy sessions. Treatment may have been provided by specialists such as rehabilitation nurses; physical, occupational, and recreational therapists; speech-language pathologists; *audiologists* (specialists in hearing); nutritionists; rehabilitative counselors; psychologists; social workers; *physiatrists*, (physicians specializing in rehabilitation); chaplains; and possibly support groups. This team approach was your first step toward meeting your individual medical needs.

Now, you are going home to begin a new phase of your recovery.

* Check with your neurologist or therapist prior to using the tips contained in this book. Have a caregiver or family member observe you until you feel comfortable performing tasks by yourself. Safety and medical supervision are of the highest priority post-stroke.

Your homecoming may seem overwhelming. Remember, your long-term goal is to be as independent as possible. Hold your head up, face your fears, and do the best that you can.

You are a stroke survivor, but I prefer the term "Stroke Hero," as the word "survivor" merely means that you have lived through serious circumstances. A hero means that we continue to live with courage and a commitment to overcoming our condition and providing a role model to others by exploring new avenues while hanging on to a positive attitude. It is not easy to be a hero while facing adversity and knowing that life is not fair. But you are a hero to your family and friends. You are a hero to other stroke survivors who will face stroke head on by looking to you for advice and finding hope in your example.

* Throughout this book, I refer to the person who has had a stroke, male or female, as a "Stroke Hero."
* I challenge you to accept the position of "Stroke Hero."

Many of the tips contained in *After a Stroke: 300 Tips for Making Life Easier* will be useful to you and your family, but you will also develop your own way of performing tasks. You will learn to push the envelope of recovery a little more each day, with safety always as your most precious guideline. Learning to live fully within the confines of stroke will be very difficult, but stroke does not define your creativity or personhood. You are a hero.

Although I have had many setbacks along the road to recovery, I have slowly discovered how to overcome them by picking up the pieces of my life and moving forward. This is called hope. Surely, there can be a triumphant and prosperous life after stroke.

During the first year post-stroke, I seemed to be a beat behind and moved to the cadence of a pathos drummer. Because I had trouble understanding language and words that were once so familiar to me, I became frantic. I began to look for sources that would ease the medical condition called *aphasia*, the loss of language skills following a stroke or brain trauma that affects the language, or word finding, center in the brain. Aphasic conditions vary. Some stroke heroes may experience difficulty finding correct words or phrases, but are able to understand what is being said to them. Another type of aphasia may cause difficulty in understanding or with reading, writing, or arithmetic. Aphasia may cause some people to lose the ability to speak. I attempted to compensate for my particular aphasic difficulties by openly tape recording face-to-face encounters in order to aid in understanding word and content meaning over time. Aphasic difficulties confused language, and I said "salt and pepper" when I meant to say "soap and water" and countless other misappropriate word choices.

* For those of you with aphasia, it is important to practice what you learned in therapy when at home, too. Try simple words that are represented by pictures. Above all, keep trying. Never give up.
* Use mirrors to help you visualize how you form words.

Further tips are included in sections called *Plateaus, Communication, Comprehension Skills, Using the Telephone,* and *Building New Connections within the Brain.* You may have had extended outpatient therapy because of aphasic difficulties. In this case, your speech therapist may have given you more tools to use as you continue to recover from your specific aphasic difficulties.

Possibly you were fortunate enough to receive a vocational evaluation that helped you acquire new skills, and you have enough energy to return to the workforce. Using this scenario, this book offers energy saving techniques that can assist you with many household tasks, cooking tips, and meditation exercises. But for the majority of readers, stroke recovery will be an arduous journey through dark and light times, tears and laughter, frustration and satisfaction, loneliness and companionship, paralysis and movement, until we reach our goal of slowly shifting from patient to person again. Let's get started.

The Basics

1. Tips About Plateaus in Recovery

WHEN YOU WERE in the hospital, you may have heard the words, "You have reached a plateau in recovery." This means that you have leveled off for a time or that you are not advancing as fast as you previously did in therapy. It does not mean you have completed the stroke recovery process or concluded making new connections within the brain.

* The first tip is that your first choice of self-empowerment is to choose to work at home, on your own and with the assistance of others, to far surpass plateaus.

Those in the medical community may say that within the first 6 weeks they project to see the greatest recovery in mobility, communication, and self-care skills in the post-stroke patient. And they work toward this goal. Your personal goal may vary from that of the stroke team. During the beginning of recovery, it is difficult to define what your actual outcome will be in the future. No one has a crystal ball, and no one can predict what many months or years of hard work on your part will produce. I have seen too many people who have had a stroke accept a plateau as an end of their recovery. Some stroke patients allow one simple word to overpower and stifle their recovery progress. They focus too much on this medical term, allowing a plateau to become a self-fulfilling prophecy by deciding they will not improve without medical treatment or continued therapy, perhaps because the word *plateau* conjures up negative images at a particularly vulnerable time post-stroke. Many plateaus will occur during stroke recovery, and stroke heroes continually exceed them.

* The next tip is to choose to believe in your power of recovery. The process will be slow and, progress is eventually up to you. But you are better today than you were yesterday, and you will continue to improve.
* If you're continuing outpatient rehabilitation, don't wait until your next session to practice what you've learned. It could be a few days or up to a week or two before your next therapy appointment. In the meantime, you and your family are in charge of practicing exercise routines taught in therapy. Brain neurons require constant stimulation in order to make new connections. It will be more difficult to progress if you depend entirely on formal therapy sessions for your total rehabilitation. No matter how fantastic your therapist is, you are in charge of teaching those brain neurons. Your therapist will facilitate by showing you the best approach.

2. Tips toward Improving Communication: Helpful Terms

THE ABILITY TO speak is extremely important in the process of stroke recovery. Relearning what, when, and how to use the language can be a challenge. How you refer to yourself and how others vocalize their view of you can be paramount to your success. You are not a victim. The word "victim" drains us of any power we may have in recovery. I am more than the stroke I had and so are you. The stroke has changed the way I perform many tasks, but it certainly hasn't victimized me. I have learned to adapt to different ways of accomplishing tasks. It may take me a little longer to perform certain acts than it did before the stroke. While you are learning how to live a full life after stroke, I discourage terms such as "stroke victim."

Another term you may hear is "good side" or "bad side" when

others refer to the use of your body. Everyone has a left and right side to his body. Although a stroke occurring on the right side of the brain may cause left-sided neglect, I still have a left side. I would not allow anyone to judge my body in terms of "good" or "bad." I had to realize that my body had a corresponding half or left side.

* I learned to refer to my left side as the "affected side" of my body and the right side as the "unaffected side." Therefore, in this book, directions and tips refer to your affected and unaffected side (regardless of whether that is right or left), to you as stroke hero, and to your caregiver as family or family members.
* A word of advice to families: We each must find our own way of accomplishing daily activities and, in so doing, realize the fruits of our labor through our own good works. Smothering us with love is positive. On the other hand, pampering us with an overabundant amount of attention and doing everything for us stifles growth toward recovery. Allow us time to heal.

I will explain in further chapters how family members can be a vital part of the recovery process, and I'll give a few tips in Section X about how *Families Need Care Too* to avoid burnout.

* As we begin to recover, remember to speak to us in short sentences. Many of us cannot assimilate long dialogs, run-on sentences, verbose questions, or multifaceted directions. We need your assistance in understanding what brain area was affected and how to best compensate for our language difficulties. Parts of these initial problems may resolve in time, but we're not sure when that time will be. Work with us as partners.
* Speak to us in your normal tone and voice inflection. We can hear the words, but may have difficulty in understanding or comprehending all that you say as fast as we did before the stroke.
* A word about choices: Our social structure has become very involved in giving consumers choices. However, too many choices may boomerang on stroke heroes, causing confusion

and frustration. For example, going to the grocery store can be an exasperating and vexing task after a stroke. The array of choices may be overwhelming, and choosing the one or two items you need may overpower you with too much sensory input, which is limited by the brain's ability to properly process or integrate information relating to what you see, hear, feel or touch, smell, and taste, and that which aids in your balance and movements. If you are looking for bread, what type? Rye, whole wheat, white, marble rye, pumpernickel, cinnamon? Do you want it sliced? Do you want rolls, buns, or croissants? And as you leave the grocery store, would you like a paper or plastic bag? "Staying focused" may be impossible directly after a stroke, or you may stay focused on something totally irrelevant, like the smell of the bread or the lights in the store. Begin with smaller grocery stores instead of mega stores. Don't avoid shopping because of sensory overload or too many choices, because you need to experience the world around you. But, be specific in your shopping request, like one loaf of sliced whole wheat bread. Instead of allowing sensory overload to overwhelm you, ask a store clerk to assist you with your purchase. Ask others to limit choices to two things. As you heal, you may be able to expand your mental list of preferences.

* Some stroke heroes, like me, have relearned to speak, but may become very talkative in the process. This may be common with a right-sided brain injury, which may affect the centers of language and speech. I became euphoric with the ability to speak again, but I did not choose my words carefully. I would jump from topic to topic in fragmented sentences and only stop speaking if I had knowingly recalled an incorrect word or phrase. I referred to this as "my brain healing on the outside for all to see." Sometimes people think, but do not speak. I had difficulty with listening and understanding, I had a delayed response that sometimes left me feeling remorseful for having possibly hurt someone's feelings. Speech therapy is vitally important for relearning speech, as

well as correct syntax. Exposure to language is important as well. Isolation leads to depression and the inability to form new neuron pathways within the brain. However, overstimulation, leads to fatigue. A delicate balance is necessary during the first few months of recovery.

* Stroke heroes may use inappropriate language, even though they never may have used such language before the stroke. A theory here is that most expletives or swear words are monosyllabic, thus easier to speak. We may say an inappropriate word, but mean something totally different. Be patient with us as we attempt to find our correct syntax again.

* Idioms and clichés, figurative speech, such as "the straw that broke the camel's back" or "that's the last straw," among countless others, may be too difficult to grasp for a new stroke hero. I would be literally looking for a camel or a straw! Our language is full of figures of speech that may be difficult to decipher in a stroke-affected brain. Use exact language. Say what you mean as we relearn connotations and nuances of the spoken and written word.

3. Tips to Assist Reading and Comprehension

IF YOU'VE GOTTEN this far in reading the book, maybe you don't need tips about reading. If stroke has affected your vision and comprehension skills, here are some helpful tools that I used to aid in relearning.

* If you have visual deficits, use a magnifying glass or enlargement reader that can be purchased through many special equipment catalogs. Check with your local therapy department or local stroke support group for magnification tools that will assist you.

* Large-print material is very helpful. Libraries offer several large-print versions of magazines and books. Ask your local librarian to supply you with large-print material.

* If you own a large-print book, draw a red line down the mar-

gin of the side of the page on your affected visual field. This will remind you to go back to the red line to catch the entire sentence.

* The National Library Service (NLS) for the Blind and Physically Handicapped has special tape recorders to lend and books on tape that will help you in auditory learning. This service is free to those who apply and qualify. Access your local Department of Vocational and Rehabilitation Services for details on how to receive this type of equipment. While you're waiting for the paperwork to be processed at the NLS, the local library may be just the spot to try books on tape and practice comprehension skills.

This service was especially helpful as I returned to college post-stroke. The Department of Rehabilitation and Vocational Services provided the financial assistance, and the NLS, through the college's Disability Services and Access Services department, supplied all text-books in the special NLS tape recorded format. Over time, this style of auditory learning, listening while visually following along with the words in the textbook, was a tremendous help in stimulating other areas within my brain to take over for stroke-damaged regions.

* Looking at the printed word while hearing it spoken will reinforce language adaptability and remind you to move your head and eyes to the end of the page to catch all the text.
* Take your time, and read one sentence at a time. Turn off the recorder or stop reading and try to visualize or slowly discern the meaning of the sentence. At first, this procedure is very time consuming and tiring. Rest. Then go back to the project when you are ready. Remember, you are building new neuron pathways in your brain.
* For comprehension skills, I used a small tape recorder and, with permission of people who were speaking to me, I taped vital conversations. In the hospital, this technique assisted my family in listening to the physician's conversation and assisted me in remembering information. In the classroom,

with the professor's permission, the system worked well to tape lectures and learn by repeatedly playing the tape.

* Remembering to use the small cassette tape player may be difficult. At first, while in the hospital, I had someone make a sign in bold letters by the tape player stating that the tape player was used for memory retention. At home and in the classroom, the tape player was the first item out of my backpack or pocket. (I prioritized everything. First, I walked to the classroom; if I got lost along the way, I'd ask someone for directions. Second, I prepared the tape for the lecture.)

4. Tips on Controlling Emotional Lability

EMOTIONAL LABILITY IS the term the medical community uses to address emotional responses that have gone awry due to stroke. However, stroke also causes strong emotional responses that are normal and natural to such physical and psychological trauma. Stroke heroes feel fear, anxiety, frustration, anger, sadness, and grief. When any loss occurs, we grieve. When a stroke hero's loses part of his ability to function, the primary response to such a loss is shock and grief. This mourning of loss was tremendously real for me in the early stages post-stroke. I mourned for the loss of function on my affected left side, the inability to communicate, the loss of comprehension, the loss of employment, and this huge, unpredictable life change, a change that I would inevitably have to make. I grieved over the loss of myself. My family grieved over their loss too.

People going through the huge emotional and physical upheavals caused by stroke encounter stages of shock, grief, anger, denial, and acceptance. We bounce back and forth between each stage until, with time, we are able to deal with this life change and work towards healing.

* Shock, grief, anger, denial, and acceptance should be addressed as part of the normal emotional responses to stroke.
* Emotional lability, such as uncharacteristic crying even

when you are happy, is a side effect of stroke and may require medication.

* Clinical depression is a sense of hopelessness that disrupts an individual's ability to function. Signs of clinical depression include sleep disturbances, lethargy, irritability, fatigue, social withdrawal, a change in eating patterns that leads to sudden weight loss or weight gain, and thoughts of suicide. If you experience any of these symptoms, consult with psychological counselors who address post-stroke depression. Antidepressant medications can be prescribed that will help you overcome clinical depression.

* If you are aware of the brain areas affected by your stroke and the functions of the affected brain regions, you are halfway to a solution.

* To solve the other half of the problem, consult with your neurologist and neuropsychologist regarding medications for medically diagnosed emotional lability or depression.

* If you experience emotional lability, know that this results from the stroke and don't be afraid or ashamed of the tears or laughter you display. Look at it this way: Your emotions may be hyperactive or overstimulated right now, but thankfully you have them!

* Your neurologist and psychologist must explain emotional lability and issues relating to depression in terms both you and your family can understand.

* Personality changes and emotional responses may be affected because you are working at understanding visual images and verbal messages simultaneously. Most people take seeing, visualizing, recognition, and emotional responses for granted. This may not be so simple if a stroke affects the visual association cortex. Nothing may have meaning. It is a frightening and frustrating experience to see an object or a person and not be able to recognize them because the knowledge center associated with identification is damaged. For some stroke heroes with this difficulty, hearing may be enhanced versus visual perception.

During the healing process, I laughed when I was saddened and cried when I should have smiled. There were also times when I had no emotional response at all. Perhaps this was due to visual agnosia, defined as an impairment to the visual association cortex of the brain. It is not because you can't see, but because you can't recognize what you are seeing. Therefore, the appropriate emotional response to visual stimuli is muted. You may be able to make out individual letters in a word, but not the entire word, or you may be able to give an accurate definition about an object, but can't recall its name. This may improve with time.

5. Tips for Differences between Anger and Rage

ANGER CAN BE a wonderful motivator, but we need to shy away from its first cousin, rage. Anger can motivate you to get out of bed to let the cat or dog out, get dressed, or even tie your shoes by yourself no matter how much time it takes to do so. Anger assisted me with not becoming complacent and accepting defeat. Anger is fine as long as it is not directed at another person or you, and it is used solely for motivation. Placing blame or anger on yourself for having a stroke is a waste of energy that you must conserve.

* Use anger wisely only to perform a single task when you are well rested.
* Make sure that safety issues are addressed before attempting the task.
* Time is your advocate, not your adversary.
* Anger can be a wonderful motivator, but its first cousin, rage, must avoid be avoided.
* Anger is a normal response; rage must be controlled.

6. Tips for Frequent Rest Periods

STROKE RECOVERY WILL not happen in a day, week, month, or year. It is a slow process that necessitates work as well as rest. You are better today than you were yesterday, and you will continue to improve as you work towards your recovery.

- Alternate exercise or activity with rest periods.
- You may tire easily, and your body and brain may demand frequent naps.
- Too much sleep may lead to depression. Intersperse rest periods with stimulating activities that challenge your concentration skills and exercise your body.
- While you work at tolerating a longer period of wakefulness, balance it with at least one nap in the afternoon.

Think of your brain as a large rechargeable battery. When it drains of power, you tire and your stroke-affected side begins to indicate the weakness. You may trip on your affected foot or droop to one side when sitting erect. Your body and brain are telling you to rest. A 15- to 30-minute nap may be enough to recharge your brain battery and keep you up and active the rest of the day. You need a "power nap!"

7. Tips for Accepting Assistance

TEAMWORK IS ESSENTIAL after a stroke. The medical personnel worked as a team while you were hospitalized. Now, your family and you must comprise the home stroke team. An encouraging cheering section does a world of good towards your improvement.

- Your attitude and effort affect your recovery process. Recovery is a lifelong process. You are better today than you were yesterday, and tomorrow you will be better than you are today. Don't give up.
- Practice as if you are learning to play the piano for the first time. You will be rewiring the electrical impulses in your brain to form new pathways.
- Challenge yourself to become creative in solving problems.
- Set realistic goals.
- Keep a journal of your recovery process. You can see how you

improve over time. Your ability to write words that gradually form sentences, then short paragraphs, will be a benchmark for your recovery. Gradually, you will see improvement in your communication skills that will encourage you to continue.

* Accept assistance from family members when you move or transfer from wheelchair to chair, bed, toilet, or bathtub, especially during the first few weeks or until you can manage safely.
* Accept the use of equipment or appliances to help you complete your transfer procedures safely. For example, a sliding board is helpful for moving between different heights.

8. Tips for Safety Issues during Adaptations

IT IS IMPORTANT that your home is adapted to meet your needs. Safety, accessibility, and independence are three main priorities. (See also the tips under Tips for Special Equipment.)

* Eliminate throw rugs.
* Always wear supportive shoes with good gripping tread soles or slippers that have safety tread soles. Beach socks are great for after a shower or bath.
* Install handrails on both sides of stairways.
* Rearrange furniture so that you can move freely in a wheelchair or walker.
* A ramp may be necessary for the steps outside your home.
* Installing grab bars in your shower or bath is always a good idea.
* Check that your doorways and hallways are wide enough to allow your wheelchair or walker easy access. Doors or door frames may have to be removed to make a wider entryway.
* Add a hand-held shower nozzle (Figure 1).
* Have medical supply companies properly install shower chairs and shower benches.
* Faucet handles that you can turn on and off with your wrist or knee may have to be installed.

* A large nonskid bath mat is essential for safety.
* Plastic pump bottles or plastic flip-top lids are easiest to use with one hand.
* A long-handled brush is great for scrubbing or scratching your back.
* A washcloth mitt or nylon puff with rope is easier to manage than an ordinary washcloth.
* Place a suction cup holder at your hand level on the wall of the bathtub for easy access to shampoo, soap, and brushes.

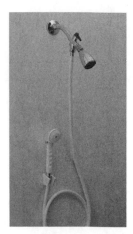

Figure 1. Hand-held showerhead.

* Don't use swivel chairs, office chairs that have wheels on the base, or chairs that are extremely low.
* Install a kitchen counter that is accessible while you are seated.
* Move items that you use frequently within your reach.

Now let's talk about appliances like walkers and canes. When you were sent home from the hospital or rehabilitation facility, you may have been in a wheelchair or using a walker or cane. You may have been fitted for a leg or arm brace or both. Your particular stroke mandates the type of appliance you need. Your neurologist, therapist, and medical team will work with you to determine what is best for your stroke deficit. In my case, with entire left-sided weakness, I used a wheelchair, then advanced to an aluminum frame walker, progressed to a four-prong cane, then a single-tip cane, and eventually I was able to walk unassisted. I wore a leg brace for several years post-stroke, and I continue to rely on it when necessary.

I broke my affected left ankle and foot several times post-stroke, and pins remain in my ankle for better stability. This is why safety issues are of highest priority: At times, you may think that you can perform tasks that actually may be too difficult for you to do safely. Falls usually result in injury to your stroke-affected side of the body. In some cases, you may not realize the extent of the injury, because the stroke has interrupted connections from the brain to the opposing side of the body.

Wheelchairs, walkers, canes, and braces are used for support, movement, and safety issues while you are recovering. Standard wheelchairs have arm, leg, and foot rests to protect your affected side. They have handles for pushing the chair, because you may have difficulty propelling the chair using your stroke-affected arm or hand.

* Your neurologist, therapist, and medical team will determine which device will work best for your particular stroke. Make sure braces fit well and check often for pressure points, swelling, or redness.

9. Tips for Special Equipment

PRIOR TO LEAVING the hospital or rehabilitation facility, you will be evaluated by your neurologist and therapist for any and all special equipment you may need. You may be fitted for aids that support your affected side and assist you in mobility. You will be instructed in the proper and safe use of necessary equipment before you venture out on your own.

Wheelchairs come in various designs and can be customized to meet your needs.

* Motorized wheelchairs have a chair for resting and a place to put small items. Aluminum frame models fold for easy transports.

Walkers provide more support than a cane and also come in different designs.

* If you have linoleum, hardwood, tile, or a floor that has a slippery surface, cut and place tennis balls on the two front leg bases of your walker. This prevents the rubber stoppers from getting stuck to the floor surface, and it makes it easier to move the walker.

* A small tray or basket can be fitted to the front of a walker so that you can carry small objects easily (Figure 2).
* Many hospital auxiliary organizations make cotton pockets that can be tied onto a walker to carry items (Figure 2).

Special beds and mattresses are also available through medical supply companies. If your physician requires you to have this equipment, she will work with you to provide the most appropriate type.

* Some special mattresses are filled with air or water and reduce pressure sores or bedsores.
* An ankle brace may be needed to provide support from the knee to the toe of your affected side. This brace is designed by therapy departments to fit your leg. It fits inside a lace-type, good gripping shoe that provides support when walking.
* An arm brace may be necessary to keep your affected arm supported and the fingers extended or bendable.
* A cane, either single-tip or with four prongs, may be used to provide balance when walking.

I used all these items, at one point or another, during my stroke recovery. Whether and for how long you will need to use these assis-

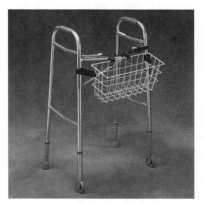 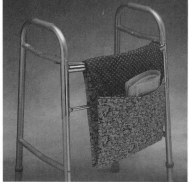

Figure 2. Baskets and cloth pouches allow you to carry small items easily.

tive devices depends on many medical factors, including your energy level. Safety is a major factor. Today, 12 years after two major strokes, I walk unassisted, but must gauge continually my level of energy. At first, I could only walk short distances without assistance. Now, my balance has improved, and I walk daily for exercise.

10. Tips for Storing and Dispensing Medications

BEFORE I GIVE tips on storing and dispensing medications, I would be lax in nursing skills if I did not mention the most important caveat of all. It seems so simple, but can be a huge task for those who have had a stroke.

* Make sure that every physician, pharmacist, and dentist you visit is aware of every medication and over-the-counter vitamin or other type of medicine you are taking.

A *contraindication* is a specific situation in which a drug should not be used, because it may be harmful. Examples of contraindications are allergies, high blood pressure, pregnancy, or the use of certain other medications. Adverse interactions can happen if medical personnel do not have a written confirmation from you or your family advising them of the names, dosages, and time intervals of your medications, and the reasons why you take them. Print this information and make a few photocopies to keep with you and/or in a notebook you take to your physician's or dentist's office. Your pharmacist is another line of defense for adverse interactions, provided that you use the same pharmacy each time you fill or refill prescriptions.

* Never purchase over-the-counter medications prior to checking with your physician; even a simple cold remedy could potentially contraindicate another medication you are taking.
* Take your medications on time and as directed.
* Never stop taking a medication unless your physician has instructed you to do so. Some medications may take time to build up in your system to work properly. Others may cause

adverse reactions if stopped abruptly. Read, or have a family member read, the side effect insert given with medications. Consult your physician or pharmacist if you have any questions about your medications.

* Place medications that don't require refrigeration in an accessible drawer with a lock that you and other adults can operate or use an old-fashioned bread keeper that can be fastened so that children cannot have access.

* Request that your medication be dispensed with easy flip-top lids versus childproof caps.

* Request bold print on medication labels.

* Some of you will take aspirin post-stroke, as an anticoagulant prescribed as a prophylactic or preventative measure to guard against further blood clotting problems. Although it is an extremely inexpensive way to possibly prevent further strokes, opening that hermetically sealed container can be difficult. Place the bottle, with cap side up, in some type of gripping device. For example, use a kitchen drawer with your body against the drawer to hold it closed or place the bottle between your thighs if you have enough power to hold it. With your unaffected hand, use scissors to cut the plastic wrapper from around the neck of the bottle. This is the tricky part. Because I have a difficult time reading small print, especially when it is the same color as the bottle cap, use the thumb or finger of your unaffected hand to feel and match up both small notches on the bottle cap and neck. Hold the bottle firmly in your unaffected hand and flip the top off of the bottle. Use tweezers to remove the cotton from inside the bottle.

* You may want to buy enteric-coated aspirin, which helps prevent stomach upset.

* Check the expiration date on aspirin bottles to make sure you have plenty of time in which to consume each tablet as prescribed. If aspirin smells rancid, it probably has expired, so throw it out and buy another supply.

* If you purchase a large bottle of aspirin, put it in your freezer

to help keep it fresh. Make sure no children can get to it! Aspirin is lethal if taken in large quantities. Take aspirin exactly as prescribed by your physician.

* If you're taking aspirin daily, as prescribed by your physician, take another type of medication for an occasional headache or to ease aching muscles. Again, check with your physician for the best remedy for pain relief. Don't take any other medication, even over-the-counter types, without first checking with your physician for contraindications.

* Once a week, set your medications up in a plastic tray that contains spill-proof flip-top lids. These medication containers can be purchased at drug stores or pharmacies or obtained through your hospital. The container should be clearly marked with the day of the week and time.

* Prepare your medications at the same time every week to form a pattern, and make sure you understand each medication's actions and its side effects.

* If you have difficulty swallowing, ask your physician for a liquid form of the medication.

* If you are taking a liquid medicine orally, use a medicine dropper or syringe without the needle. Your pharmacist will be able to provide you with one that is clearly marked with amounts. Using you unaffected hand, draw up the required dosage into the dropper or syringe, and then take the medicine. Make sure all medicine bottles are closed securely after every use.

* If your medication is to be taken with food, make sure you place a reminder on the pillbox. For example, place a mark that will remind you to eat. If you are to take the medicine on an empty stomach, place another simple symbol on the lid of the medicine box to remind you to take it between meals.

* Make sure you take your medications with you if you are going out for the day or on a trip.

* When traveling, carry your medications in your purse, waist belt bag, or backpack, along with an emergency card containing your physician's name, contact number, and a list of

all medications you are currently taking.

* Never pack medications in your luggage. The luggage may be checked at an airport, for example, and become lost, or you may miss taking your next dose.

* If you are diabetic, you must travel with the equipment needed for checking glucose levels, along with your medication. Small packs can be purchased through your local pharmacy for diabetic care and insulin storage while traveling.

* Make sure you have water available when taking medications.

* If you have difficulty swallowing, tuck you chin to your chest when attempting to swallow. Sometimes, pills can be ground up and taken mixed with a soft food that makes swallowing easier. But check with your physician or pharmacist first, because some medications may need to stay in their original form for proper absorption.

* Remember, sometimes stroke heroes get sick too. If you catch a cold or other virus, your affected side may become weaker than usual while your body internally fights the virus. Make sure your physician is notified if you become ill.

Getting Ready

1. Tips for Personal Care

AT FIRST, YOU will find that personal care seems awkward when performing tasks one-handed, and each task may take an extremely long time to accomplish. In time, and with a few helpful hints, these tasks will get easier and more familiar to you. Be creative. Take time to think about how you can perform familiar tasks in a new and easier way.

* Plan your actions before trying to perform the task.
* Then perform each task one at a time until it gets easier.
* Discover what works best for you.

2. Bathing or Showering

IT IS MUCH safer to take a shower rather than lower yourself into a slippery bathtub. It is more difficult for your family to assist you out of the tub than out of the shower. Here, we address safety procedures and hints for both bathing and showering

* Locate everything you need within easy reach before you get into the shower tub. This includes liquid soap in an easy-access plastic bottle, a mesh netted bathing puff, a combination shampoo and conditioner in one easy plastic applicator, a long-handled brush, and a towel.
* An elongated scrubber that has grab loops at both ends works best for scrubbing your back. These are available at most

shower and bath shops; they have terry cloth on one side and a rougher texture on the other side. Loop the scrubber over your affected fingers, placing the loop between the thumb and palm. Place the scrubber over your shoulder and grasp it with your unaffected hand. This technique also works well in moving your affected arm and hand. Gently, gently, gently, use your affected arm and hand as ballast.

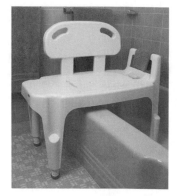

Figure 3. Bath and shower chair.

* Make sure you have a large bath mat with suction cup grippers or a nonskid surface in the tub or shower.
* Test the water temperature with your unaffected hand prior to getting into the shower or tub.
* If you are taking a tub bath, place a towel on the side of the tub. With the assistance of a family member, sit on the towel and use the same technique as you do in getting in and out of a car: Place your unaffected foot in first, use a wall-attached grab bar to hold onto with your unaffected hand, and lower yourself carefully into the tub.
* Medical supply companies sell shower chairs or tub seats that can attach to the side of the tub (Figures 3), but you may need a family member to assist you in getting out of the tub.
* A helpful hint I used immediately post-stroke was that, after my bath, I let the water drain out of the tub and dried myself off in the tub before attempting to climb out. As long as the bathroom stays warm and you don't get chilled, this technique works quite well. Use the grab bar to assist you in standing up, and then sit on a towel draped over the edge of the tub. Swing your unaffected leg over the edge of the tub, followed by your affected side. Make sure you have assistance and that the tub and floor are dry.

* An adjustable bath transfer bench, with or without back support, is much easier for showering.
* While seated safely in the shower, take advantage of this opportunity to exercise your affected arm. Try shoulder rolls, then hold your affected hand with your other hand and gently guide your affected arm to bend at the elbow. Knead your affected fingers with your unaffected hand. This will be difficult at first, but you will be providing sensory input.
* Wash your affected side, including armpit, with liquid soap and the mesh netted bathing puff by holding onto the looped strap on the puff with your unaffected hand. Another trick is to use a short-handled dish-washing sponge.
* Hand-held shower heads make it easier to reach to wash your hair, underarms, and private areas.
* Use large absorbent terry cloth towels. Sometimes two bath towels sewn together or slipping on a comfy terry cloth robe works well to dry you off after a bath or shower.
* You can wash your hair with your unaffected hand.
* Special attention should be taken while washing and rinsing your affected side. Touching or lightly rubbing your affected side with your unaffected hand during bathing is a very positive step toward your re-awareness that it is, in fact, part of you and you are stimulating brain neurons to acknowledge the affected side.
* Apply body lotion after your bath to prevent dry, chafed skin. This is a great time to observe body parts for pressure, swelling, or redness. While seated, squeeze or pump body lotion on parts of your body using your unaffected hand. Rub it in and observe ankles, feet, and other areas for skin breakdown. Make sure you rub lotion into your affected hand too. Move as much of your affected hand as possible with the assistance of your unaffected hand for tactile stimulation. Even though you may have no sensation in your affected hand, moving it as much as possible improves circulation and may help movement.
* To apply deodorant, lean forward and let your affected arm

dangle away from your body, then reach in to apply deodorant. Another technique is to lift the affected forearm and hand as far up as possible and bend your head to place your affected hand on top of your head to hold it in place. Both techniques require practice. The second technique requires the ability to move your affected arm.

* Toenails should be clipped after bathing, while they are soft and pliable. The unaffected foot can be done by placing it up on the side of the tub or something sturdy. However, your affected side is more difficult to reach and see. Until you have recovered enough to place your affected foot over your unaffected knee to comfortably reach your toes, it is advisable to have a family member clip the toenails on your affected foot. If you are diabetic, consult your doctor for special foot care procedures.

* Always check fingernails and toenails on your affected side. When toenails grow too long, they can cut into your toes on your affected side without you being aware of it.

3. Adaptive Aids

MAKE, BUY, OR procure only the equipment you need for your present adaptive lifestyle. You may improve in time and find a task easier if performed in another way. As you recover, you may become less and less dependent on adaptive aids. In some cases, you may need them, but in other situations, you may call upon your own problem-solving skills. By creatively solving problems, you are working the brain as well.

Safety is always of greatest concern, and bringing thought processes to a proper conclusion may be difficult early in your recovery. Your brain is rewiring as new connections are forming around the damaged areas, and they need input from you regarding what to do. Trying to make your life easier while at the same time trying to get your affected limbs working to some degree will be a constant balancing act. The Boy Scout motto, "Be prepared," is also appropriate for stroke heroes. Some items of clothing, kitchenware, and equipment that I have found extremely useful are:

* Elastic waistbands on slacks, pants, or skirts
* Velcro™ closures on shoes, shirt cuffs, or blouse cuffs
* Coiler shoelaces (Figure 4) that can be pulled closed but do not need to be tied
* Elastic shoelaces
* Button hooks
* Zipper jackets with string or an easy plastic breakaway tab (Figure 5) attached to the end of the zipper for easier reach and closure
* Sports bras that fit over the head or front closure brassieres
* Tube socks (without a heel)
* Large magnifier
* Rocker knife or knives (Figure 6)
* Rolling cart (Figure 7) for easy food preparation and to hold commonly used utensils
* Cutting board with suction cup feet and spikes and a vise grip for safely and easily slicing, dicing, mincing, or chopping food (Figure 8)
* A jar and can opener that you can use one-handed (Figure 9). Several styles to choose are available from adaptability catalogs
* A pizza cutter and cheese cutter, because both items have a

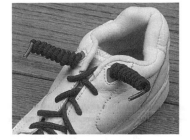

Figure 4. Coiler laces allow for one-handed tying.

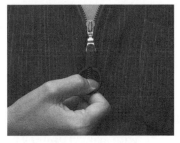

Figure 5. Zipper pulls make dressing easier.

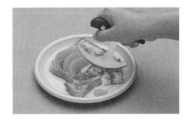

Figure 6. A rocking knife allows you to cut food easily.

variety of uses

* Wall-mounted grab bars
* Long shoe horns
* Tongs of various types; long-handled salad tongs, ice tongs, or anything that is fastened together and has a large gripping surface and good hand support
* Pullover shirts and sweaters that are a size larger than you normally wear
* Earrings that have metal wires that snap into a back fastener are easier to fasten than post earrings.
* Place your watch on the wrist of your affected side. I use a leather band type with a buckle and place the watch dial on my wrist, flip my wrist over, and lay it on a flat surface and buckle it with my unaffected hand. When I want to see the time, I must learn to be cognizant of my affected arm.
* You will need assistance putting on T.E.D.® (thromboembolism disease) stockings, because they fit tightly against the leg to prevent swelling. These stockings are part of the daily uniform for most stroke heroes. Make sure

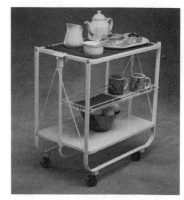

Figure 7. A wheeled cart helps at mealtimes, and also has many other useful purposes.

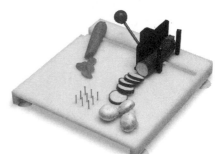

Figure 8. A cutting board with steel spikes and a vise holds fruits and vegetables for easy cutting

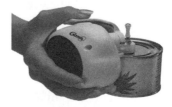

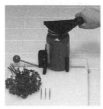

Figure 9. One-handed can and jar openers.

you wear them, especially when you are traveling in an airplane, because the inside cabin pressure can cause severe swelling in your affected leg.

4. Tips for Transfers

A TRANSFER MEANS to safely move your body from one location to another. Most people who have had a stroke learn transferring techniques while in the hospital or rehabilitation facility under the guidance of qualified therapists. Make sure a family member or caregiver has practiced with you and your therapist so that you both feel comfortable performing transfers when you are at home.

An *assisted transfer* works using this technique:

* To begin, make sure you are as close as possible to the place you are transferring or moving to. Place both chairs and transferring points at an angle if possible.
* Make sure you are wearing shoes and your leg brace, unless you are being assisted to the tub or shower.
* For the first few months post-stroke, wear a leather belt through trouser or pant belt loops so that an assistant or caregiver can hold onto you safely.
* If you are transferring to or from a wheelchair, lock the brakes and remove or move any footrests prior to attempting any transfer procedure.
* Plan the transfer procedure with your caregiver before it is carried out. Talk out the steps.
* Move as close to the edge of the seat as safely possible. Support your weight on your unaffected side as much as you can safely.
* Caregivers should bend and lift with their knees, not with their backs.
* While transferring, stand close to your caregiver assistant, with feet slightly apart in a firm stance.
* Your assistant should reach under your affected arm and lift you by grasping your belt. Stand and balance. Now, pivot toward the new transfer site. Reach back with your unaffected

hand and grasp the armrest. The caregiver can gently lower you to the new transfer place by again bending at the knees and keeping the weight evenly distributed.

An *unassisted transfer* should be undertaken only after you and your therapist feel that you are capable of performing such a task.

* Make sure your shoes and leg brace are securely fastened before beginning.
* Move to the edge of the chair seat. If you are using a wheelchair, make sure the brakes are on.
* Stabilize your weight on your unaffected foot. Lean forward in a crouched position and hang onto the chair's armrest. Boost yourself to a standing position. Pivot your body to the new chair or transfer spot, hold the armrest for balance, and lower your body into the chair.

Your therapist will teach you about other transfers as well. Some of these techniques will include transferring in and out of a car, and transferring to and from the toilet, tub, shower, bed, or other uneven transfer surfaces. Learn the safest and most comfortable way to transfer for your limitations. Be sure that your caregiver knows your transfer technique and feels comfortable in providing necessary transfers for you.

Figure 10 shows a swivel cushion for easy transfers in and out of cars.

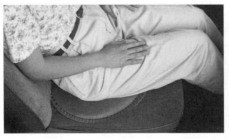
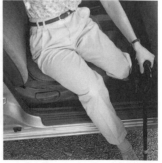

Figure 10. A swivel seat pad assists in getting in and out of a car.

5. Tips for Dressing and Undressing

YOU HAVE KNOWN how to dress yourself ever since you were a child of two or three years. So, why is the task so difficult after a stroke? It is because the area affected in the brain has injured some of its connections. This is a very simplified answer to a complex situation that has occurred within the brain, but with practice, you can learn to perform some of these basic skills once again.

* Lay out all the clothing you will wear the next day the night before. Think of clothing next to your skin, underwear and socks, and then outer clothing like shirt, pants, and shoes. Another way to remember is to start at your feet and work up. You need shoes and socks, pants and underwear, shirt, and bra or T-shirt. I use a mnemonic such as UPSSS to remember underwear, pants, socks, shirt, and shoes.
* Undress your unaffected side first and clothe your affected side first.
* Establish a routine of getting dressed every day so that you will feel better about yourself as you progress from patient to person again.
* It will be easier, and much safer, to dress and undress in a sitting position, rather than trying to balance while standing.
* For women, pullover, front closure, or sports bras may be easier to put on than regular back-closure bras. If you have a back-closure bra, you can hook it closed by putting it on backwards. Then turn it around on your body, place your affected arm into the bra strap, followed by the other arm, and lift each strap up individually. When removing the bra, use the opposite procedure. Slide the strap off the unaffected shoulder and slip your arm out. Then slip your arm out of the strap of your affected side. Turn the bra around and unhook the clasp.
* If your affected side is on the left, it may be easier to wear men's shirts that have large buttons, because they close in the

opposite direction.

* Large buttons are easier to manage than small ones.

* Shirts that have buttoned wristbands are extremely difficult to button with one hand. If you purchase a blouse or shirt of this style, try it on prior to purchase and make sure the wristband is large enough for your hand to fit through with the buttons closed.

* Blouses with small buttons can be slipped over the head with only one or two buttons unfastened, as if it were a T-shirt, and then the two buttons can be fastened. Put the sleeve on your affected arm first. Place your unaffected arm in the other sleeve and slip it over your head and down your body. The blouse must be large enough to accommodate this movement when buttoned.

* Pantyhose are a nuisance for most women who have had a stroke. Only wear them when absolutely necessary. They're difficult to put on and take down and pull up for toileting. Thigh-high nylons are not good for leg circulation problems. Wear the T.E.D.® stockings when you are in one position for an extended period of time, as when traveling in an airplane or a lengthy journey in the car. It is best if someone assists you with putting on these elastic stockings. Pantyhose and elastic T.E.D.® stockings should be gathered up between the thumb and fingers of your unaffected hand and placed on your affected leg first. While seated, place your toes into the stocking toe piece. Pull the gathers until the heel is in place. Tug gently on each side of the stocking as you slowly pull it up the leg. Repeat the same procedure on the unaffected leg.

* Shoes that have Velcro™ fasteners are best. Shoes that have sturdy, thick rubber soles and come up high on the instep give better support and may stay on you affected foot better. Some of these styles include loafers, shoes that zip closed on the instep, bear-claw sandals, boots, or walking shoes that can be laced with self-closure type laces.

Because of balance and left-sided weakness, I am unable to wear any type of high heeled shoes. Shoes that provide support and are comfortable, especially on my affected foot, are more important for safety and movement than are fashionable, pointy high heels. I would rather wear simple style shoes that I can manage alone and feel comfortable wearing than give in to chic-styled shoes and end up back in the hospital with a broken ankle.

* Your leg brace may be fitted into a shoe with good support. The shoe may be a size larger than you usually wear. When you purchase shoes, you may have to buy two pairs to compensate for the brace. Shop at shoe outlet stores that offer two pairs for the price of one!
* Mittens versus gloves: I live in the northern part of the country where winters are harsh, the snow is deep, and the layered look is protocol. You may prefer to wear a mitten on your affected hand and a glove on your unaffected hand. If you opt for the mitten look, be sure the cuff pulls up far enough to stay on your affected hand. I wore mittens during the first winter post-stroke, but worked off-season?during the spring, summer, and fall?at learning to put a glove on my affected hand. The problem with this is that I can't feel my fingers, especially when they're inside the glove where I can't see them, so I have to fish for each finger to work it into the glove. This takes time, patience, practice, and determination and is a positive step towards manipulating your affected fingers.
* Remember, you may not feel the cold on your affected side, but your fingers, as well as all extremities, are subject to frostbite. If your unaffected side is cold, properly clothe your stroke-affected side too.
* In the winter, "bundle up," as mom used to say, and wear thick tread boots. Pull-on type boots are the best choice.
* Always have someone with you when you go outdoors in the winter because under most of that snow is ice. Ice and stroke heroes don't go well together unless that ice is in a glass.

6. *Tips for Nail Care*

* If you are diabetic, consult your physician regarding your specific foot care procedures. After a stroke, it is extremely important that you do not cut your own toenails, because circulation issues may be compromised.

* If you are not diabetic, it may be difficult to perform nail care and foot care on your stroke-affected side because of visual, balance, and dexterity difficulties. Don't let the nails on your affected foot grow too long for proper shoe fitting and walking.

* When you can afford to do so, get a professional manicure and pedicure at a shop specializing in this service. Not only does a professional service solve the difficulty associated with nail care, but it provides opportunities to practice talking on the telephone, making appointments, arranging transportation, and conversing with others.

* Keep your fingernails and toenails short, smooth, and equal on both sides of your body.

* Soak your toenails in warm water to soften the nails before cutting and filing. A luxurious foot soak using a deep plastic dishpan of warm soapy water placed on a towel while you are sitting in a comfortable chair can provide relief as well as be a beauty aid.

* To clip your toenails, make sure you are in a comfortable and sturdy chair and bring the foot you need to access across your opposite thigh or prop it up on something stable at knee height.

* Clip your toenails straight across with a nail clipper. Check your stroke-affected foot for sores, swelling, or chafing, especially between the toes. Apply lotion and rub it in thoroughly. Change socks daily. Wear clean socks made of cotton or other material that affords breathability.

* It may be difficult to file the fingernails on your unaffected side with your affected hand. Place an emery board on a rectangular, well-sanded block of wood that has a groove cut into it. Then, gently file each nail separately. Someone with carpentry skills can easily make this block of wood for you.

✻ Nail care is a great time to manipulate your stroke-affected hand and foot with your unaffected hand. Observe and move each finger and toe separately to make sure each area is in your field of vision. A magnifying device or large mirror may assist with this task. Observe, carefully stimulate, and care for your affected side.

7. Tips for Shaving
(Men, face; Women, legs and underarms)

✻ It may be easier for both men and women to use an electric shaver after a stroke. For safety, this may be the best route to take. However, I found that an electric razor aggravated the thalamic pain or central nervous pain experienced on my affected left side. The second choice is a disposable safety razor. The blades do not have to be changed, and they are inexpensive.

✻ When using a disposable razor, a man en can apply shaving cream or foam to the back of his affected hand and use his unaffected hand to apply the cream to his face.

✻ Be very careful shaving the affected side of your face (for men) or affected underarm or leg (for women). The task will become easier with time.

✻ Men should make sure that a large mirror and good lighting is available to see all aspects of the affected side of their face. After shaving, feel the affected side with your unaffected hand for any areas that you may have missed.

✻ For women, shaving your stroke-affected underarm during a shower or bath may be very tricky. I had difficulty holding the disposable razor and shaving the unaffected side with my affected hand. When shaving the affected underarm, lean forward and let your affected arm dangle away from your body, then reach in to shave. Another technique is to lift the affected forearm and hand as far up as possible and bend your head to place your affected hand on top of your head to hold it in place. Both techniques require practice. The second technique requires the ability to move your affected arm.

* To shave the unaffected underarm, tape a disposable wooden tongue depressor blade (as are used in the doctor's office) to extend the handle of a disposable razor. Use your unaffected hand to reach your unaffected underarm to shave.

8. Tips for Hair Care

* A short hairstyle that can be maintained using styling mousse or styling gel and a hand-held hair dryer may be the most practical during stroke recovery.
* Use a large hand-held mirror to observe the back of your hairstyle. With your back to the bathroom mirror, look into a hand-held mirror. You may find that wall-mounted mirrors, which also tilt to a magnifying side, very useful. Remember though, that a wall mirror must be mounted on the wall of your unaffected side and remember to push it closed after every use to avoid bumping into it.
* A wall-mounted hair dryer that can be used while perched in its position will allow you to style your hair while drying it.
* Apply a small amount of styling gel or styling mousse to the back or palm of your affected hand and then apply it to your damp hair. Rub it in, then use the blow-dryer and styling brush.
* If you have long hair, make sure it stays in place and out of your face by attaching a wide barrette or hair clip at the nape of the neck with your unaffected hand.
* Curling irons or curling brushes can be used in the same way as a hand-held hair dryer. One very important caution here is that the stroke-affected side of your head may not feel heat. Be very careful not to get too close to the scalp with heated brushes or hot curling irons.

9. Tips for Dental Care

* After a stroke, you may be tempted to use your teeth for assistance, rather than your affected hand. Do so with caution.

Dental work is extremely expensive. Some things should not be placed in your mouth. Also, you will be forming adaptability practices that will circumvent the use of your affected side.

* Make sure to attend regular dental appointments and alert your dentist to your stroke, especially prior to teeth cleaning or dental surgery. Sometimes, premedication must be given if you have a heart condition that warrants a prophylactic precaution.

* A cordless electric toothbrush works well for teeth cleaning, tartar control, and gum stimulation. Also, it helps make your teeth feel as if you've just visited the dentist for a cleaning.

* A one-handed disposable flossing pick can be used easily after brushing or to remove food particles.

* Toothpaste or gel can be applied to the toothbrush when the brush is placed on the counter and the paste is applied to the brush with your unaffected hand. If this is difficult, apply a small amount of paste to the back of your affected hand and scrape it off onto the toothbrush.

* If you have dentures or a dental plate, after soaking in a cleaning solution made especially for dental devices, clip the denture into an alligator clip (a tie clip-like device) that has been affixed to a sturdy and secure block of wood so that the denture is upright and secure. Then, brush your denture, rinse thoroughly, apply adhesive if necessary, lay the block of wood containing the denture down on a counter, and unfasten from the holder. Insert the denture or plate with your unaffected hand.

The Greatest Strength Comes From Within

1. Tips for Improving Self-Esteem

THIS SECTION ADDRESSES a philosophy of stroke survival that has assisted me during 12 years of stroke recovery. I hope that you will find some useful tips toward your recovery too.

Over time, I have developed a mnemonic for the word stroke. A mnemonic is a device, code, or technique that assists memory. I have assigned a word to each letter in the word STROKE; each word represents important meaning for stroke heroes during the healing process.

* **Strength** encompasses an attitude that admits that, on the one hand, life isn't fair, but on the other hand, challenges empower us to broaden our perspectives. We have the power to change the way we look at things. We can be enthusiastic and full of hope toward finding new ways of accomplishing goals, or we can choose to complain and pity ourselves into the depths of depression. Sometimes, we get overwhelmed if we try to do everything alone, because the process of recovery requires a team and family approach. At times, we may need help from our physicians, in the form of antidepressant medications that ease the personality changes and emotions often associated with stroke. We must choose to surround

ourselves with people who love us, and in their presence, we can admit our vulnerabilities. Admitting that we are not superhuman is such a wonderful and freeing experience. This acknowledgment allows us to fully enjoy the simple pleasures in life. Strength also means that, although we continue to face challenges that change our direction, and even more so—our bodies and minds—we cannot change the past. Our power lies in our reaction to the challenges we face every day.

* T stands for time to heal, evaluate, and learn about yourself and your particular medical condition. There is no simple answer to when or how fast you will improve. But you can begin to process information as a chemist does in a lab, one very small step at a time. Research and learn about your particular stroke-affected areas. Question and try new and innovative techniques in stroke rehabilitation. Set small goals and work towards them each day. Keep a journal or record of your progress. Break paradigms rooted in misconception about stroke and your recovery. Become an advocate for other stroke heroes.

* Rehabilitation is an ongoing commitment that does not stop when we are discharged from the hospital or rehabilitation unit. Instead, hospital terminology takes on new meaning in our lives. Physical therapy evolves into performing daily exercise at home. Vocational therapy means learning new skills and learning to perform our daily tasks in a new way. Occupational therapy triggers the use of the Department of Vocational and Rehabilitation Services to help us devise new ways of accomplishing our goals. Recreational therapy becomes our community involvement. Finally, emotional therapy means family education, which is needed so that others understand our medical condition and the world around us. All of these medical aspects of stroke recovery are ongoing as we slowly move from being a patient into being a person once again and as we learn to adapt to a new lifestyle.

* Opportunity means that sometimes we have to knock on many doors to make changes occur. But among the many

challenges we face are opportunities for spiritual, educational, and personal growth. Think of the many things you wanted to do, but never had the time to do before. For example, there may be an opportunity to enhance a hobby or special interest by contacting the Department of Vocational and Rehabilitation Services in your area. An opportunity for spiritual or religious growth happens quickly when we face medical and emotional challenges. Seek your spiritual leader or religious affiliation for advice and direction. Stroke is a humbling experience. Yet, this life-changing event brought me closer in tune with my spiritual self. Also, there are opportunities to learn by flipping your stroke deficits into stroke assets. Instead of thinking of what the stroke has taken, think of how you can enhance what you have. I use a calculator rather than adding or subtracting numbers in my head, because my particular stroke has affected the portion of the brain that recognizes and remembers mathematical computations. Adjustments are difficult at any age, and under the circumstances of stroke, alterations in lifestyle can be extremely difficult. Every facet of your life may become modified. You may need to call upon new strategies and innovative skills. Be patient, keep a healing journal, stay focused, and show your love every day.

* Knowledge and kindness means being kind to yourself and to your loved ones. Family dynamics require understanding. Relax, regroup, and take one task at a time. However, be careful not to stifle recovery with too much kindness. There is a great difference between allowing stroke heroes to learn new tasks on their own and overprotecting them. Finding the balance between safety issues, time constraints, and allowing for the independence of each family member can be problematic. Slow down and modify your lifestyle to involve individual problem solving. The team approach that started in the hospital must include the family. Your family unit will become your greatest advocate.

* Environment means that safety is of ultimate priority.

Uncluttered and well-organized space allows room for the concentration of thought processes. Tools to work body and mind may involve some type of daily exercise, easy crossword puzzles, and coins for counting. Coins can be used to develop small muscle coordination as well. Try picking them up from a flat surface and placing them into a container. Always have paper and pen available for writing, drawing, or as a communication aid. Most important, environments include the people we love, respect, and rely on to help us heal. We have much to offer them too. Everyone thrives on love. We can turn stroke deficits into assets when we stop labeling people and address husband and wife, or couples, equally. Your environment definitely includes your partner.

2. Tips for Foraging through Financial Fallout

MEDICATION, FOOD, AND housing are the three basic necessities after stroke. The outdated basic needs—food, shelter, and clothing—just don't seem to complete the picture after stroke. Prescription costs are of paramount concern; if you don't get your medications and take them as prescribed, all else is irrelevant.

* Tell your physician if you are having difficulty in purchasing your medications. An open dialog with your physician is the first step in making sure you do not go without your medication. Your physician will refer you to programs that may assist you.
* Check with pharmaceutical manufacturers about receiving their program guidelines regarding how to get their products at low cost or on a sliding fee basis.
* Never go without your medication, and always take it as directed. Too many people hoard medication and take it improperly, saying, "Half is better than none." Your medication will not work properly if not taken in the amount prescribed, when prescribed.

Your ability to provide an income may change. You may be faced with the financial burden of mounting medical bills. If you were considered high-income before the stroke, you may be able to afford private in-home therapists and care assistants. Perhaps you won't have to worry about sorting through medical charges and stressing over who owes what to whom. But for the majority of us, get ready for a bewildering brawl between insurance companies and numerous medical providers. Here are a few tips for shaking that money tree:

* Check with your place of employment for any disability insurance policies that you may have paid premiums for and that may benefit you now.
* Check your homeowners or mortgage insurance policy to see if you carry disability insurance that may assist with mortgage payments.
* If you have a home, keep it. Have it adapted to fit your needs. Your home is sheltered from most creditors. Utilities for your home are part of your housing cost and will be appropriately factored into most supplemental programs for which you may qualify.
* If you have a mortgage with no disability insurance, you may want to call your mortgage company and arrange for an alternative payment schedule. Telephone or write your mortgage company and request information on refinancing at a lower interest rate. If this is not possible because of increased interest rates, check the term of your mortgage. You may have to renegotiate the contract. This could mandate new closing costs, but these costs could be absorbed within the new mortgage. Ask if you can take your 15-year mortgage over a 20- to 30-year period instead, if applicable. The mortgage company may like the idea of collecting more interest, and you may feel more comfortable paying less money each month. Remember, your mortgage interest is tax deductible.

Your savings may become depleted. Even with an excellent medical insurance policy, you may reach the "maximum insured benefit coverage," at which point the insurance company is no longer obligated to pay for your health costs. Getting another company to insure your health may be impossible, as you now have a "preexisting condition." The only alternative may be Medicare and/or Medicaid (if over 65) and the limited options offered under these programs. Options are limited because, once you've had a stroke, you must choose the program with the maximum amount of coverage.

Medicare does not pay for prescription costs, and this fact continues to cause controversy on a national level. The discount card advertised through Medicare only applies to low-income patrons. This discount program allows for a limited $6,000 in benefits in 1 year and limits the monthly amount of medication coverage to $600. Even if you are low-income, you will be responsible for paying anything over that amount when picking up your medication from the pharmacy.

The financial picture may be bleak. Your spouse's income (if applicable), along with any savings or individual retirement accounts (IRAs), could be your only source of expendable monies.

* Check with Veteran's benefits (if applicable) or any other type of retirement benefits connected with long-held employment.
* Ask your physician if you should file for Social Security Disability Insurance (SSDI) benefits.
* If you do not have enough actual work weeks paid into SSDI, ask a social worker to assist you in applying for Social Security income (a program that assists low-income citizens).
* When and if you are considered disabled by Social Security, you may withdraw your IRA funds without penalty for early withdrawal.
* When you have received your acceptance letter from SSDI, you may apply through your state property tax assessor's office for disability status for homesteaded property tax. This Disability Homestead Tax Credit will decrease the amount

owed on your property taxes as long as you are disabled. The verification must be completed annually.

In time, you may be able to work from your home or on an extremely part-time basis outside the home.

- As you improve, begin to work with the Department of Rehabilitation and Vocational Services in your area. This governmental agency can assist with education and job training towards a new vocation.
- The Red Book is the Social Security Administration's booklet that explains how you can attempt to work while continuing to receive SSDI benefits. It is a complicated system of weeks worked, monthly income received, and possible annual physical reviews.
- Some states offer Medical Assistance benefits if you are employed. This state-operated program is income-regulated. But if you benefit from SSDI, you may be able to qualify for Employment for Disabled People (EDP) as well. On this program, you pay a sliding fee amount for this insurance per month. Medical Assistance will be a secondary medical insurance carrier to Medicare. However, Medical Assistance-EDP will cover your monthly medications with a very small amount of co-pay from the recipient. Medical Assistance-EDP also pays for the monthly cost of maintaining Medicare, so the entire amount of SSDI you are entitled to goes directly to you.

Of course, many other financial and personal care matters must be addressed. For example, will your medical insurance cover home health assistants, in-home therapy, equipment, housekeeping help, or food delivery services such as Meals-on-Wheels? Does your pharmacy provide delivery service or can a family member pick up medications when necessary? Have you recovered enough to be left alone while your spouse or other family members goes out to work?

✽ Remember the basic requirements: medication costs first, food and dietary needs second, and housing third.

Citizens must demand improvement in government-operated Medicare, SSDI, and especially the affordability of prescription medications. However, it is extremely difficult to be in the position of demanding anything when you are aphasic or while working on overcoming other severe difficulties post-stroke. When we are healthy, we don't think about advocating for these issues. But when we lose our health and ability to produce an income, we are suddenly faced with the reality that there may be no lifeline.

Given few alternatives, some citizens and state programs (for example, Minnesota) attempt to control their prescription costs by purchasing medications from Canada. As health care costs continue to rise, and to keep up with cost overruns in this supply and demand economy, Medicare premiums are on the increase. When an individual's household budget is limited to monthly disability benefits, it may be impossible to meet the swelling costs of health care, medications, food, and housing.

I would be doing you a disservice if I tried to paint a rosy picture or ply you with positive platitudes about your personal finances. As someone who has foraged through stroke fallout, I am able to address the general concepts of long-term disability issues and give you a few options. Everyone's financial picture will vary. But the three basic needs will remain constant: medication, food, and housing.

3. The No-Joke Stroke or How Humor Helps Heal

THERE IS NOTHING humorous, funny, cute, or comical about stroke. Instead, depression is an all too common symptom. Stroke is the leading cause of long-term disability and the third leading cause of death in the United States, according to the American Heart Association\American Stroke Association and the National Stroke Association 2003–2004 statistics.

Friends or family may try to get you to smile or laugh by telling a joke or a humorous anecdote, but because of comprehension difficulties, you may analyze every word literally and, in the process, lose the amusing meaning. Language is more than words; tone, pace, expression, and innuendoes also make up communication.

But humorous incidents happened to me post-stroke—even if it took me a few moments to catch on. When I finally understood, I could hardly stop laughing, not only because of the humor, but because I realized I *understood* the humor. I understood abstract thinking instead of just concrete terminology. I got it!

* Within a year or so after the stroke, I returned to college. In the classroom, I was so intently focused on taking notes, listening to the professor, reading the chalkboard, and following the lecture that I didn't notice my spastic stroke-affected left arm. That arm, my arm, began to swerve and wave in the air as if it had a mind of its own. The professor called on me because, surely, I must have a question with my hand waving in the air like the flag on the Fourth of July. I looked around, obviously perplexed at his attention. This went on relentlessly, until I realized, by looking to my affected side, what I was doing. I started to laugh and, by doing so, gave permission to the entire room to break out in thunderous guffaws. I told them that I had just washed my hand and couldn't do a thing with it! From then on, I remembered to put my affected hand under my thigh during class. The students were not laughing at my disability. They saw humor in the inappropriateness of raising a hand in class and having the professor stop lecturing to answer the question, only to realize that the student didn't have a question at all. It was humor at its finest, but no one could laugh until I broke the ice.
* When you are able to comprehend humor, you are definitely healing.
* When you are able to laugh at your own foibles and faux pas, you are on the right road to recovery.
* Carol Burnett said, "Comedy is tragedy plus time." For a stroke hero, humor is tragedy turned upside down.

I have a friend who had a stroke, and we trade humorous healing idiosyncrasies. During his stroke recovery, he was preparing his boat for its maiden launch by painting it. He climbed into the fishing boat, sat down in the middle seat, and started painting. He painted everywhere he could reach, except for where he was sitting. When he was finished, he had painted himself inside the boat! I don't know if, at the time, he saw the humor in the situation, but years later, he still relates the story of the time he painted himself inside a boat.

* The adage "When you fail to plan, you are planning to fail" applies to all of us.

Sometimes humor lies in the infinite planning we must do to accomplish a task. I could easily call my neighbor to change a light bulb in a ceiling fixture, but I like to be as independent as possible. It took me 2 days to devise a plan that took into account safety and my permanent stroke peccadilloes of vertigo, left-sided weakness, and fine motor deficiencies in the left hand. I took the trusty cordless phone with me on this expedition in case I'd have to call for assistance halfway through the task, I wore a vest that contained a hairnet, strips of masking tape, the new light bulb, and of course the phone with preprogrammed numbers for immediate dialing. I wore a sturdy wide leather belt with another belt slipped through the first with an S-hook clamp fastened to the buckled end. I climbed an expandable solid wooden ladder like a rock climber, and with each step, hooked the S-hook onto the other side of the ladder for stability. When I could reach the fixture, I hooked the S-hook on the far side of the top of the ladder. When leaning forward on the ladder, the light fixture was on my unaffected side directly above me. I removed the fixture cover screw, palmed it in my unaffected hand while holding onto the light fixture, and carefully placed the light fixture on top of the ladder. I taped the hairnet to the ceiling on three sides over the burned out bulb. Then, I unscrewed the deficient bulb and allowed it to fall into the makeshift net. I replaced the bulb and took the net with the used bulb off the ceiling and placed it in my vest pocket. After replacing the light fixture cover, I kept it in place with my head until I could pull the nut up from my hand to my fingers and screw it in securely. Remembering the S-hook, I unhooked it and hugged the ladder while I climbed down one step at a time. All the while I tried to stay focused, but couldn't help thinking about warnings such as, "Don't do this at home" and jokes like, "How many stroke survivors does it take to change a ceiling light fixture?" The answer, dear reader, is just one and a lot of creativity!

* When you plan too much, the task may seem overwhelming.

Humor serves as a great healing tool. I have laughed at my 18-hour bra, aptly named because it usually takes me that long to put it on! I have laughed at the patient gown I don while watching the Academy Awards. The actresses' designer gowns may have hefty price tags, but my cotton hospital gown with the slit up the back cost approximately $1 million in total medical care. And I am worth every penny. My gown may be more expensive than the actresses' designer dresses, and I use my gorgeous gown during speaking presentations as an example of the tremendous cost of stroke care.

* Love yourself. Your medical team worked diligently to get you this far. Surprise them, yourself, and your family with what you can do independently.
* Practice smiling. Others will wonder what you're up to or at least what kind of medication you're on!
* A stroke hero related to me that "life has become a tactile sport" regarding his visual impairments and memory difficulties. By touching objects, he is able to recall the name of them.
* In my case, wishing for a BMW has been replaced by merely hoping for the first two letters, in order to function normally.
* Laugh when things strike you as humorous. Laugh at your ability to laugh. Laugh at your insight to grasp abstract humor and keep that feeling close to your heart. Your brain is mak-

ing new connections. You are healing.

* Here's a humorous healing tool that also shows how the right and left hemispheres of the brain work to control the opposite sides of the body. Sit down and make clockwise circles with your unaffected foot. At the same time, using your unaffected hand, draw the number 6 in the air in front of you. Your foot will unconsciously start moving in a counter-clockwise motion.

Let's Get Cookin'

1. Tips to Improve Mealtimes

MEALTIME SHOULD BE a quiet time because you must concentrate on the procedure involved in eating: preparing small bites of food, placing them on a fork or spoon, chewing, and swallowing. Things that we did not think about prior to stroke must be planned in painstaking order now. Distractions such as eating in a noisy restaurant or lively table conversation may cause problems while chewing or swallowing food properly and lead to choking. This swallowing difficulty following stroke is called *dysphagia*. (The word *dysphasia* refers to a cognitive loss of ability to understand, speak, read, and write.) Consult your doctor if you experience swallowing or choking difficulties.

* Wash your hands thoroughly before eating or preparing food.
* Don't try to answer questions, carry on table conversation, or listen attentively while you are eating. Your focus should be on the act of eating. One activity at a time is appropriate after stroke.
* Take small bites of food.
* Eating utensils may be easier to grip and hold in your hand when accentuated with a larger soft surface (Figure 11).
* Tuck your chin into your chest when swallowing small amounts of liquid or food to prevent

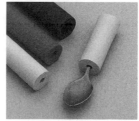

Figure 11. Large, soft grip handles for utensils.

choking.

* Sometimes liquids may need to be thickened with an additive provided by your therapist or physician to assist swallowing.

* Soft foods or foods processed in a blender or food processor may be easier to swallow without choking than bite-size pieces of food.

* Check for trapped food in the affected side of your mouth after every bite.

* Use utensils that are easy to hold. Those sold through adaptability catalogs are longer, allow for a wider fork plate, and have padding around the handle.

* Chew food on the unaffected side of your mouth.

* Containers, such as butter, cream, sugar, and milk cartons, are difficult to open with one hand. Place the small individual butter container in the palm of your affected hand. Steady the tiny container with your affected hand. Position your affected thumb over the container and pull the tab with your unaffected fingers. If this procedure is too difficult for you, grip the container or packet between your teeth and pull across with your unaffected fingers. Sugar packets can be placed in front of you or secured partially under your plate with your unaffected hand. Tear the sugar packet open at one end and remove the packet with your unaffected hand.

* Why fight with trying to open small objects while at a restaurant? Ask the server to open creamers, butter containers, sugar, or whatever condiments you use all at once and to place them within easy reach on your unaffected side so that you can see them. Don't forget to leave a nice tip for this added service.

* If you are at a restaurant, remember to hold the menu on your unaffected side so that you can see the entire fare. Order food that is soft and easy to eat to avoid choking. Request the food, especially meat, cut up in small pieces when ordering. Restaurants will provide this service for you, and you will feel more independent. If you have a visual impairment, make sure you turn or rotate your plate to see

food on your affected side or move your plate over within your visual field.

2. Tips for Cooking

I LIVE BY the motto: "As ye cook, so shall ye clean." If we stay clean up as we go, it won't be as difficult. So let's get started.

* Line the counter around your stainless steel-spiked cutting board with newspaper for easier clean up.
* When using a recipe, gather all the needed ingredients first and then place a pencil mark on the recipe after adding the ingredient or finishing the step. This process helps you stay on task.
* Peel carrots, potatoes, or any vegetable by stabbing them onto the spikes on the cutting board. Make sure the suction cups are secured to the counter for a firm grip. See **Figure 8.** pg 44.
* Slicing and dicing can be easily accomplished using a food processor.
* Slice and dice by hand by using the vise grip on your cutting board to hold a vegetable while you use a rocking knife. Different types of rocking knives are available.
* Make sure your knives are sharp and that your affected hand and fingers are well out of the way. A wall-mounted knife sharpener works well for one-handed sharpening.
* When using a large cooking pot, fill a smaller pitcher or measuring cup with the liquid you need and pour it into the pot after it is on the range top. Absolutely avoid trying to carry hot or bulky items to or from the stove!
* Stirring or mixing with one hand can be difficult, because the bowl or pan spins around if not anchored. Stirring ingredients in a bowl can be accomplished three ways: 1) Place the mixing bowl in a top drawer of your kitchen cabinet and close the drawer around the bowl to secure it. 2) Sit back on a chair and place the mixing bowl between your knees. 3) Use a non-skid pad material (Dycem) that fastens to your counter and the bottom of the bowl (Figure 12).

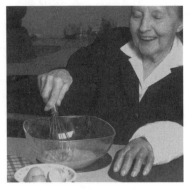

Figure 12 A. A nonskid pad makes food preparation more comfortable.

Figure 12 B. Dycem® nonskid material can be cut as needed.

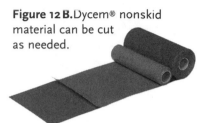

* Stirring a pot on the front burner of the stovetop can be easily managed by anchoring the pan handle against another heavier pan on the back burner. Place the first pan's handle at the counterclockwise position against the heavier pan and stir clockwise.
* To place or remove items from the oven, use a long-wristed padded oven mitt. If the item is too heavy to lift with your unaffected hand, ask for assistance.
* Microwaves are lifesavers for defrosting frozen meats and heating up leftovers or a quick bowl of soup, cup of coffee or tea, popping popcorn, and preparing foods. Use the recommended timing for your microwave, because accidents can occur when you overheat liquids and then attempt to stir them. Allow covered liquids to cool in the microwave for a few minutes before handling, pouring, or drinking them.
* Flip-top cans may be easier to open than cans that do not supply a ring to grasp. Use the tip of a small butter knife or another utensil that has a long, flat edge, to pry the ring up a bit for easier reach. Place the can in the vise grip of your cutting board or grasp it between your thighs when in a sitting position. Using your unaffected hand, grasp the ring, and roll your hand close to the lid, prying the top off away from you.
* Opening a can sometimes requires a can opener that can be operated with one hand. I use a hand crank can opener. First, I pierce the can with the opener in my unaffected hand. Then

I switch hands and stabilize the opener with whatever grip I can get with my affected hand and turn the crank with the unaffected fingers. This provides exercise for my unaffected hand. A cordless hand-held opener is much easier for one-handed use.

* Open jars by first tapping the top rim with the handle of a butter knife or placing the rim under warm water to loosen the vacuum. Then, place the jar between your thighs while you are seated and place a rubber mat over the jar lid. Hold the jar in place by gripping your thighs together as much as possible and twist on the rubber mat with your unaffected hand.

* When setting the table, use nonbreakable dishes, cups, and plastic glasses. I always keep a cardboard six-pack carton, of the type sold with soda bottles or beer, as a simple caddy on the table. It holds folded napkins and silverware and even makes condiments easily accessible.

* Plastic containers with seal-tight lids or zipper-type storage bags work well for refrigerator food storage. Get the air out of a zip-type bag by laying it flat on the counter, then placing your affected forearm above the food, on the outside of the bag. With the air released and holding the bag secure with your affected arm, zip the bag closed using your unaffected hand.

* You can become proficient at cracking an egg with one hand. Try it over a small bowl first, to prevent eggshells from getting into your recipe. Palm the egg gently in your unaffected hand, turn your hand over, and crack the egg on the side of the dish. Quickly move your hand over the bowl and separate the eggshell by lifting up with your thumb and small finger.

* Purchase food already partially prepared or cut into individual portions, such as boneless and skinless chicken, for easy portioning and preparation.

In addressing cooking skills, it is also important to talk about the food you may be preparing. After a stroke, your energy level is decreased. You may lose weight in the hospital, but after being at home for a while, you may gain weight. This may be due to lack of exercise and because you are unable to perform your regular routine. Follow you physician's advice regarding your diet at home and check with a dietician if you are diabetic or need special dietary requirements.

Because being overweight is prevalent in American society, you must be vigilant about controlling your weight to prevent an exacerbation of other disorders, like heart disease.

I have read many books on the subject of dieting and tried several types of diets. But measuring food, counting calories, and studying the small print doesn't seem to work for me. I have trouble keeping track of mathematical calculations and find it impossible to read small-print packaging labels. After bouncing between hunger and weight loss to eating voraciously and gaining weight—the yo-yo approach to dieting—I found it necessary to make a permanent lifestyle choice. I settled on a Southern European, Iberian, or Mediterranean menu. This type of food was instilled in me by two PhDs in cellular biology from Portugal who live with me for an extended period each year. We share meals, grocery shop together, and collectively prepare food. During this eclectic living arrangement, I have the opportunity to explore new foods and incorporate new eating habits.

* By eating small meals six times a day (breakfast, morning snack, lunch, mid-afternoon snack, supper, and evening snack), your stomach is always full.
* By avoiding fast-food restaurants, your wallet gains weight and your heart stays healthier.
* By using olive oil, a monounsaturated fat, to cook with and on salads, you avoid unhealthy polyunsaturated fats.
* Eat fresh fruits and vegetables and low-fat yogurt or cheese every day. Fresh fruits and vegetables are rich in antioxidants, and antioxidants are compounds that prevent the oxidation of molecules in your body. These compounds may be useful in delaying the aging process and in preventing diseases, such as some forms of cancer and heart disease. Antioxidants may also help reduce the extension of ischemic lesions in the heart or brain caused by a stroke or heart disease.
* As opposed to a low-carb or no-carb diet, I choose to eat fresh

breads, rice, potatoes, or pasta daily. Carbohydrates quickly turn into sugar within our body, so diabetics must control their intake of carbohydrates. But, if you are on a regular diet and meal plan, your body uses carbohydrates quickly through exercise. Of course, "carbo-loading" is only necessary the night before a high-energy long-term event, such as a marathon run. Anything in excess is contrary to your body's require-ment. Carbohydrates are a necessary source and mainstay of the Southern European or Mediterranean style of eating.

* Eat small amounts of fish and chicken, or other types of poul-try, several times each week; eat red meat as a treat only occa-sionally.
* Fresh cooked eggs can be eaten two or three times each week.

By controlling hunger and eating six small meals a day, I have experienced a great improvement in my energy level and have been able to control my weight as well. The tiny cup of espresso that is the traditional dessert at the end of a Mediterranean style meal is something that I usually forgo, because I am sensitive to caffeine late in the day.

Once in a while, I waver from this eating style, especially when I am away from home. But when I return, I go back to my Southern European style of eating.

* Try to limit caffeine products, especially in the evening, because caffeine may interrupt your sleep patterns. Juice, water, and decaffeinated iced tea are good substitute beverages.
* Red wine, in moderation, may help you sleep. However, exces-sive alcohol may cause a headache.
* Exercise regularly, regardless of your diet. Regular exercise is vitally important, especially for stroke heroes. I walk. I keep good muscle tone and posture by moving my body through space. Stroke recovery is a "use it or lose it" proposition.

Washing and Drying Dishes

* Use a long-handled scrubber or other dishwashing device,

available at most discount stores.

* To hold dishes while washing them in the sink, line the sink bottom with a nonskid pad.
* Use a dish drainer in both sinks, as well as on the draining rack, to hold items steady while you wash and rinse. Place one item at a time into the dish drainer.
* As you prepare a meal, rinse, wash, or place in the dishwasher the dishes, pots, and utensils you use as you go, so that you will have more counter space to maneuver.
* Presoaped pads that come several in a dispenser work well for washing dishes with your unaffected hand.

3. Tips for Cleaning

I HATE HOUSEWORK, but it's got to be done. So let's get started.

Laundry

If your washer and dryer are located in the basement, beware because there's a terrible hazard between you and the appliances — the stairs.

* Make sure hand railings are installed on each side of the stairways. If you use a walker, cane, or wheelchair, you cannot safely navigating this obstacle.
* Don't attempt to use the stairs until you are instructed by your therapist on the proper technique to use, when appropriate.
* Never use the stairs without someone there to assist you or to call for help if necessary. Never use the stairs without a portable phone in your pocket.

If you are able to climb stairs but tire easily, here's my approach to basement stairs.

* With a portable phone in a pocket or short apron, I sit down on the top landing. I hold onto the railing with my unaffected hand and place my feet on the third step. Then, I ease my

body to the first step and repeat the procedure until my feet are on the floor, and then I stand up.

* To go back up the stairs, I hold onto the railing with my unaffected hand and take one step at a time, followed by the affected foot: I stand, balance, move my hand up on the railing, lift my unaffected foot up another stair, and repeat.
* Make sure the stairway is closed in on both sides or has solid handrails on both sides.
* Stairways should be very well lit. Always turn on the light.

Once you have reached the washer and dryer, here are some tips to making laundry easier:

* Most people can sort clothes and operate a washer and dryer with one hand.
* Tie a rope or long belt through the handles of a small laundry basket so that you can carry it more easily or drag it if you have to.
* Never overfill laundry basket.
* Use a roller cart to move full laundry baskets around.
* Sit down to sort or fold clothes.
* To fold sheets, bath towels, and other large items, lay the item on a table top, place the top two ends together, and smooth it straight. (Make sure you have the correct ends together on the correct side so that it isn't twisted.) Fold the end together again. Straighten out this end first, then move down the item, following the pleats and folding over as you go.
* Smaller items are easier to fold than larger ones, but don't get discouraged. Someone can always help you do the folding sheet dance, and you can use your unaffected hand and your opposing elbow and body to assist you with this partnered two-step.
* Match socks and fold in half together as a pair.
* Forget about being a perfectionist! I do the best I can with folding laundry, then place the folded laundry on a wheeled cart and pull it around, placing the clothes in their appro-

priate drawers or linen closet.

* Use the Joan Crawford rule in the movie Mommy Dearest and never use wire hangers. Not only, as my mother said, will they "poke your eye out," but they're hard on clothes. Use plastic or cloth covered hangers that you can purchase at discount stores.
* To save on wrinkles and ironing, hang up pants, slacks, shirts, and blouses as soon as they're finished drying or allow them to dry on the hanger.
* To hang pants, grab the bottom of both legs and shake them so that they are not twisted. Lay the garment on a long table or ironing board. Put the four seams of the pants together and shake the pants again by holding onto the seams with your unaffected hand. Lay the cuff or bottom of the pants over the hanger. Slide the hanger to the middle portion of the pants and pick it up. Your pants or slacks are ready for the closet or to be line dried. To hang T-shirts, place the plastic hanger up from the body of the shirt to the neckline. For a blouse or shirt, button the top button while the shirt is lying on the table facing you. Then insert the hanger and hang the shirt or blouse up; adjust the shoulder seams on the hanger with your unaffected hand.
* Make sure you empty the lint filter in your dryer after every load. Pull the filter out with your unaffected hand and brace it on the dryer with your affected elbow, arm, or hand if possible, or put it between your knees. Roll off the lint with your unaffected hand. Replace the clean filter.
* Vacuum behind your dryer every once in a while, too, to prevent fires.

Polishing Furniture

* A long-handled, lightweight magnetic duster works well for high places like the tops of draperies or ceiling fan blades.
* A dusting mitt works well for tables and low areas. Some mitts come with polish already in the fabric of the mitt. Polish

and toss the mitt away.

Vacuuming

* A lightweight vacuum cleaner that you can handle is much easier than one you have to tote around.
* Wind the vacuum cleaner cord loosely around your affected arm to make sure you don't trip over it as you vacuum.
* Small hand-held vacuums work great for little messes, and they can be snapped into their recharging holder on a wall for easy access.
* When using a full-size vacuum cleaner, stand in one spot and push it back and forth in front of you. Then, take a couple of steps and repeat the process. When finished, plan a strategy for not tripping on the cord. Turn off the vacuum cleaner, place the handle upright until it snaps in place, and gather the cord around the cord holder as much as possible. While holding the cord line out away from your body toward the electric receptacle, follow the cord with your unaffected hand until you can disconnect it.
* If you use a walker, it is difficult to balance and vacuum at the same time. Remember, safety first! Try negotiating a compromise with your partner. Maybe your partner will vacuum if you dust or fold laundry.

Sweeping the Kitchen or Bathroom Floor

* Sweeping with one hand is easy if you position the broom handle across your unaffected shoulder and grab the broom lower down on the shaft.
* Purchase a long-handled dustpan, position it against a wall, and place one foot

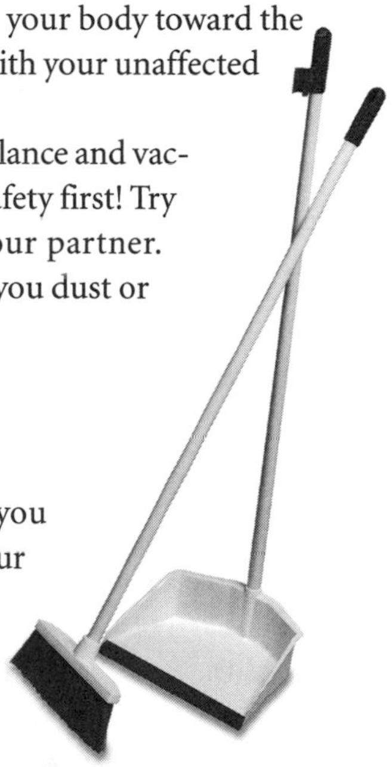

Figure 13. Long handled dustpan and broom set.

on the dustpan opening. Now it is stabilized enough to provide for sweeping into the pan (Figure 13).

Mopping or Scrubbing Floors

* Instead of scrubbing floors on your hands and knees, you can sit on the floor and scoot along, scrubbing as you go.
* To clean floors almost effortlessly, purchase a handy all-in-one system that holds a bottle of cleaner inverted on a mop handle with a disposable mop pad head. You change the mop pad after every use by pushing in four prongs. I prop the handle against my body, dispense the liquid, and then mop the floor.
* Once a month, I revert back to a routine of sitting on the kitchen floor and scrubbing the floor the old-fashioned way with a bucket of cleaner and a scrub brush. By using this method, I can get those areas I may have missed by mopping. I scrub as far as I can comfortably reach, then scoot or push my body to another spot and complete the task. If you use this technique, make sure you have practiced with your therapist the safest way for you to get up to a standing position. I have a very small kitchen floor and scoot to reach the sink counter for support. Never use a movable piece of furniture to support your body.

Making Beds

* Use contour sheets and try to make one side of the bed at a time to save energy.
* To change bedding, pull all the bedding off one side and roll it as tightly as possible over to the other side of the bed. Then, place a fresh contour (bottom) sheet over the mattress pad on one corner and make sure it's tucked under the mattress at the head of the bed. Pull it down and do the same for the foot of the bed. Bunch the rest of the sheet in the middle of the bed. Put the top sheet and blanket on. Stretch the contour sheet around the bottom of mattress so that it does not flip off the opposite corner while you stretch it over the other corners of the mattress. Tuck the top sheet under the mattress, using

the fingers of your unaffected hand. Once you have finished the bottom and one side of the bed, go to the other side of the bed and remove the soiled linen by balling it up and placing it out of your way. Pull the bottom contour sheet over the top of the mattress first. (It is easier to pull the sheet onto the bottom corner of the mattress when you do not have a footboard in the way.)

* Square corners can be made at the bottom of the bed, but it is difficult to hold the mattress up while tucking the sheet or blanket underneath. (A hint: If you are steady on both feet, lift the corner of the mattress up, tuck your knee underneath the mattress, and wedge your foot on top of the box springs.)
* Sit down to replace pillowcases. Hold a corner of the soiled pillowcase on the floor with your unaffected foot and pull the pillow out. To put a fresh pillowcase on, bunch or gather the pillowcase first, put the pillow in the end, then pull the gathers out on each side.
* Use an all-in-one comforter, which is much easier to smooth across the bed than blankets and a bedspread and doesn't require tucking in.

Moving Furniture

THIS IS A HIGHLY controversial issue. Do I advocate that all stroke heroes move furniture as a part of home therapy? No, I do not. If you can get someone to move the furniture for you, by all means, use brain instead of brawn. I have cajoled, bartered, and formally requested household chores of neighbors, contractors, and friends. The trick is to know your capabilities. But I also advocate for as much independence as safely possible post-stroke. I include this section because in time, you may want to move something heavy. Many years after my stroke, once I was able to walk without the assistance of a walker or cane, I decided to move the furniture around—including a heavy oak upright piano! This is how I did it.

* When placing furniture on carpeting, use special plastic disks that make it easier to move and save on carpet indentations

as well. These disks are available at most furniture stores or discount stores and go under each leg of heavy items. However, make sure someone strong enough to lift heavy furniture puts the disks in place for you.

* First, before moving anything, sit down and plan your attack. Where should you place the furniture for convenient access? What strategy is involved in moving the large items?
* Second, move or drag smaller or lightweight items out of the way, such as small end tables, chairs, lamps, coffee tables, or portable a television on a wooden wheeled stand.

After I did these preliminaries in my own home, I was ready to tackle moving the piano:

* After making a large enough path to move a big item from point A to point B, clear off any items that might be on top of a large piece of furniture, including removable sofa pillows, art objects, removable drawers, and the like.
* If a piece of furniture has wheels (as my upright piano did), make sure all four wheels are turning in the same direction. This may call for a tug on one furniture leg, or it may require you to get down on the floor, eye level with the wheel and manipulate it with your unaffected fingers.

To move my heavy, wheeled piano, I used my body as a lever. I sat down against the wall, braced my unaffected leg against the piano leg, and moved it a few inches. Once my body could fit behind one side of the piano, I used my unaffected leg and sturdy soled foot to move out the other side. Turning the wheels again in the direction I wanted the piano to move, I leveraged my unaffected side against the piano, and bent my knees in a tucked position, so as not to injure my back. Then, I budged it a couple of inches and rested.

It took a long time to move the piano from one wall to another because I rested so often between leveraging it with my torso. I knew I could not drag it or pull it without injuring my back. Pushing along the smooth side of the piano seemed to work well as long as

I was crouched down and pushing with the unaffected side of my entire body and using my legs as leverage. Another strategy I used was to lie on the floor on my back with my legs bent and push on the side of the piano with both feet.

Although I do not recommend moving a piano post-stroke, I mention it because I want you to realize that the impossible is sometimes possible given time, patience, and careful planning.

After moving furniture (or doing any heavy exercise), it is a good idea to assess your body for damages. Stand in front of a full-length mirror completely naked and examine yourself, especially your affected side. Look for bruises, scrapes, or other signs of injury.

4. Tips for Carrying Things

- Use an apron or hunting vest with several pockets to carry lightweight objects.
- Practice carrying using an empty, lightweight, unbreakable foam cup in your affected hand and walking a few steps. Gradually move up to attempting to carry an empty paper cup, empty pop can, or other nonbreakable item.
- Purses with long straps that can be placed over your head and across your body or small fanny packs that can be snapped around your waist are great, because they allow for hands-free carrying. Canvas bags with long straps are great for toting things too.
- Pouches can be made or purchased for the backs or sides of wheelchairs for easy access.
- Practice carrying an empty nonbreakable plate, napkin, and utensils in preparation for the dreaded buffet line.
- At a buffet dinner, refreshments are usually served at the table, but if they are not, only fill your glass halfway when attempting to carry it in your unaffected hand and sit at a table close to the buffet.
- Never carry coffee or hot items. You may be unfamiliar with the surroundings; people may be moving about and talking, causing distractions; you may bump your affected side; or

you may spill the hot item on your affected side and not realize or feel the scalding effect. Do what you are able to do and request assistance when needed.

* Grocery bags with handles are good for carrying lightweight items. Be careful not to overload a paper bag or it will break. Fold clothes or laundry and place the items in grocery bags to carry between rooms.

For four years I did not have access to a car, so I had to improvise new techniques for required grocery shopping. The grocery store was within walking distance, but carrying more than a small bag of groceries was beyond my capabilities. I purchased a folding cart at a local discount store.

* Lightweight, wheeled, folding carts are easy to tow along behind you when folded and, when expanded, they provide a deep narrow basket for carrying three to four bags of groceries. These inexpensive carts are extremely handy anywhere in the house too: You can load the cart with laundry and detergent for trips to the laundry room or use it for a variety of other household needs.

5. Tips for Home Maintenance

YOU'VE HAD A stroke, but if you own a home, you probably would like to keep the equity up by performing seasonal maintenance. If you live in a climate that changes from warm summers to freezing winters, you're probably wondering how you will ever be able to keep up on house maintenance chores. Sometimes it takes a little cunning: Many times, I have been accused of acting like Tom Sawyer did in getting the picket fence whitewashed. I have made statements like, "It sure is a nice day for climbing up on that ladder and looking at the view. Oh, while you're up there, could you clean out the gutters?"

If a task is beyond your capability, ask for assistance.

* Check with your physician first, before attempting any home

maintenance chores. Start gradually until you build endurance. Rest frequently and take your time.

As a homeowner, you have the same responsibilities as any other homeowner: The winter demands shoveling snow, autumn leaf raking, spring and summer grass mowing, gardening, and cleaning out rain gutters. I do call a truce at climbing ladders, and I get someone to do the rain gutter cleaning job. Let's begin with summer and lawn maintenance.

Summer

* A cordless electric lawn mower works great. I keep mine plugged in all year-round when not in use. When the lawn needs mowing, I disconnect the power and snap in a safety starter. By easily moving a lever on the handle, the mower starts. If I need to stop it, I just release the handle. Mixing gas and oil can be complicated and pulling a cord to start an engine usually takes coordination and strength. I opted for a cordless electric style that is easy to use.
* If your yard is large, mow the lawn in sections. For example, mow the front yard one day and the back yard the next day. Remember not to mow during the hottest part of the day and to drink plenty of water to keep hydrated.
* Use a long-handled manual weed trimmer instead of an electric or gas operated weed whacker.

Autumn

* Raking leaves uses the same principle as sweeping the floor with a broom. Do it one-handed by holding the rake with your unaffected hand and resting the handle against your shoulder. If you want to switch positions, use your affected hand and arm to stabilize the rake and pull with your unaffected hand.
* Rake the leaves onto a large tarp, gather the sides together, and drag small amounts at a time to garden beds to mulch them for the winter.

Winter

Snow shoveling can be difficult for anyone. I have not attempted operating a snow blower because of safety issues. Instead, I shovel. During a winter storm, I try to keep up on the snow by shoveling often while the snow is light and fluffy. If it becomes too difficult or nightfall prevents keeping up with snowy weather conditions, I, like everyone else, wait until morning. At times, I have been faced with mountains of snow so deep I can hardly find the driveway or sidewalk. These winter storms mandate calling the local snowplow service for help. A neighbor with a snow blower is an added bonus during winter storms.

If the snow is light, and you can manage walking with good, heavy tread boots and lots of warm clothing, try using a lightweight shovel with a broad base to push the snow in strips across your driveway or sidewalk.

Lifting a shovel filled with snow may be difficult. Take your time; affix the shovel handle under the arm of your unaffected side and leverage the shovel using your unaffected hand.

The dreaded end-of-the-driveway ridge caused by the city snowplows can be tricky. If ice is under the snow, be extra careful. Use a smaller shovel with a long, narrow base and take a small amount of snow at a time. (Using this smaller shovel, I widen the driveway by cutting down the snow piles on each side of the driveway, to make sure I can see traffic when backing the car into the street.)

Spring

Rain gutters need cleaning in order to maintain proper drainage away from the house foundation or windows. Tools are available to clean gutters while standing on the ground, but I have found them difficult to operate with one hand. Climbing an extension ladder or foldout ladder is not recommended for stroke heroes with one-sided weakness and/or coordination or mobility difficulties. A hose with a long extension that can be affixed to a sturdy pole may work, but I have found that trading favors with neighbors works much better. I barter washing their car for cleaning my gutters or washing a few reachable windows on their home for their assistance with difficult chores. Knowing your limits will prevent accidents and cement neighborly relations.

Painting

The kitchen needed a fresh coat of paint, so I gathered all the necessary tools and a gallon of semi-gloss paint and asked the neighbors to come over for a painting party. I fired up the gas barbeque grill, made chicken and a large potato salad, and provided a nice lunch. Voila! The kitchen had an entirely new coat of paint in no time at all. If the house needs painting, try the same procedure, but work along with your friends to scrape and paint what you are able to reach. Do what you can do best and ask for support when necessary.

Let's Mention Unmentionables

1. Tips for Controlling Urinary Incontinence

THE BRAIN CONTROLS the voluntary and involuntary movements and reflexes relating to urination. Normally, we feel an urge to void and respond by using the bathroom when we need to empty our bladder. However, when a stroke affects brain areas related to the urinary process, we may become incontinent.

* Don't despair; the problem may resolve itself in time.
* Limit the liquids you drink in the evening hours.
* Use the bathroom every 2 to 3 hours whether you feel you need to or not. By using this procedure, you allow time for your brain to heal and you offer your bladder frequent relief.
* Set a timer or alarm to assist you with remembering this routine.
* Use the bathroom before going to bed and directly upon awakening.
* Set an alarm clock to wake you during the night to remind you to visit the bathroom or have a commode or urinal close to the bedside for easy and quick use during nighttime urgencies.
* Place a waterproof protector between the sheet and mattress pad of your bed in case of accidents.
* Some medications may cause urinary frequency. Check the inserts on all prescribed and over-the-counter medications you are taking for side effects and consult with your physician.

* If the problem does not resolve within a few moths, check with a urologist, a doctor specializing in the urinary system.
* Clothing that has elastic waistbands makes it easier to use the bathroom.
* If necessary, disposable undergarments can be purchased to protect outer clothing during this healing phase.
* Keep your skin clean and dry to prevent chafing, irritation, bacteria that form odors, and possible bladder infections.
* Lack of exercise, inadequate liquids during the day, and improper diet can lead to bladder problems. Activity, nutrition, and liquids that do not contain caffeine assist urinary control.
* Contact your physician if you notice any signs of a urinary tract infection that complicate your stroke healing process. Signs of infection may include fever, burning upon urination, frequent urination, cloudy urine, or blood in the urine.
* Use a raised toilet seat cushion that can easily be fastened to standard toilets for ease in toileting. These cushioned seats can be purchased through an adaptability or medical supply store (Figure 14).

Figure 14.
A padded, raised toilet seat.

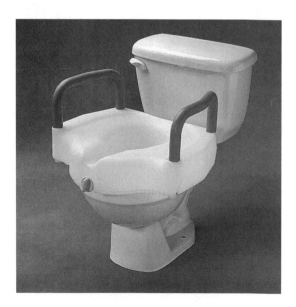

SECTION VI

Let's Get Moving

1. Tips for Using the Telephone

IT MAY BE extremely difficult to use the telephone post-stroke. If you have any type of aphasia, it may be even more challenging, but you may be able to get special telephone typing equipment, such as a telex system, or a picture phone through the telephone distribution center listed in the Resources section of this book.

* One alternative may be a *hearing carry over* (HCO) system, such as the one offered through Minnesota Relay. This system allows a hearing person without audible speech to place a telephone call through the relay system with help from a communication assistant. The HCO user types her words into the device, and the communication assistant reads then reads the message to a standard telephone user.
* The Telephone Equipment Distribution (TED) Program provides telephone equipment to people who are speech impaired or have other physical disabilities and need adaptive equipment to use the phone. Equipment is loaned out at no cost as a long-term loan. Several types of equipment are available, including hands-free speakerphones. To learn more about adaptive equipment available through the TED Program, have a family member or hospital therapist check with your local Department of Human Services office. The TED Program is offered in every state.

Remembering seven numbers, even if they are written down,

while trying to find the matching number on the telephone, is sometimes exhausting. But communications systems have come a long way over the past few years. Today, special equipment is available to prevent being isolated from the world while you are healing from the effects of stroke. The following are some ideas I used when my speech improved enough to use the phone.

* Use an answering machine to filter calls and to keep track of necessary information.
* Practice phone calls with family members first. This technique will assist you with voice modulation and listening skills.
* Purchase a telephone with large numbers on the keyboard, preferably one that is hardwired, that is, with a cord from the receiver to the push-button numbers. This will assist with one-handed manipulation, because you will be able to put the receiver in your lap as you press the numbers on a stable surface. Then, pick up the receiver with your unaffected hand.
* A family member should request that your telephone carrier offer you free directory assistance because of your disability. It may be too difficult to see the small print in telephone books or find the number in a large book.
* Always have paper and pen or pencil ready by the telephone (Figure 15).
* When calling directory assistance, request that they give you the number personally rather than through their automated system. Repeat the numbers, one at a time, as you write each one down. If this is too difficult for you, ask a family member to get the phone number for you.
* When dialing an organization, agency, or corporation that has an automated answering system, dial "0" to get an operator as soon as

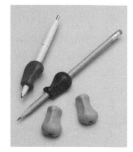

Figure 15. Soft, slip-on grips make pens and pencils easier to use.

possible to avoid being barraged with complicated instructions. These systems are becoming more common every day and are extremely difficult for many of us to navigate—too many instructions and too much talk may cause you to forget why you telephoned, or you may not be able to comprehend all the instructions. Ask a family member to make the phone call for you after you have explained or written the purpose of the call.

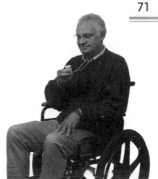

Figure 16. A necklace type personal pager provides greater security.

* Keep frequently called numbers in a notebook by the telephone. Make sure they are written in large print.
* Keep phone conversations as short and uncomplicated as possible.
* Tell your caller that you need information in short simple sentences or to send you the information via mail.
* Keep a portable or cell phone with you, especially if you use a walker or cane. In case of a fall, you can reach assistance. Preprogram the portable phone so that you can dial emergency services or a family member with the single push of a button. Make sure you understand how to seek assistance if necessary. If you dial 911 but cannot speak due to your stroke, an ambulance will be summoned automatically, so just stay on the telephone line.
* If necessary, use a personal first responder system for safety (Figure 16).
* A phone in the kitchen and next to the bed, within easy reach, is necessary for safety.

2. Tips for Mobility

* If your balance is unsteady, make sure a therapist evaluates you to ensure what type of mobility aid is best for you.

- Request an evaluation of your home as well. A therapist can assess your needs and make specific suggestions toward modifications that could simplify your daily living.
- Don't rely on wobbly furniture to support you while walking. Chairs may tip or move and place you at an awkward angle for support while walking. Use your walker, cane, fitted brace, or wheelchair for support.
- Make sure you never overload your walker bag or tray with heavy items, because this may tip the walker and cause you to fall.
- When shopping, use the motorized carts provided by many stores. They are usually stationed at the front of the store.
- Ask your physician to authorize a disability parking permit for your car. You can get a disability tag or license plate from the motor vehicle department in your area. Use the disability parking spots near building entrances to reduce walking distances, especially in inclement weather.

3. Tips for Car Transfers

- Open the car door as wide as possible.
- If you are transferring from a wheelchair, bring the chair close to the car and station it at about a 90-degree angle to the car seat. Station the chair between the car door and the car seat you will transfer to.
- Lock the breaks on the wheelchair.
- Hold the door frame for support to assist you to a standing position, pivot toward the car seat and sit down sideways, then swing one leg at a time into the car.
- Buckle your seat belt. Reach up for the shoulder harness with your unaffected hand and snap it into the fastener under your unaffected arm by your waist. If your right side is the affected side, reach up with your left hand and pull the shoulder harness down and snap it into place. Ask for assistance if necessary. In any case, make sure you are buckled in before traveling in any motor vehicle.

* When getting out of a car, unsnap the shoulder harness, pivot or swivel your body toward the open car door, and swing one leg at a time out of the car. Hold onto the open door frame or an assistant for support, and transfer to a wheelchair or stand erect with walker or cane.

* If you have an assistant, have them wrap their arms around your upper body and bend at the knees to help you stand. Be sure to bend your head slightly to avoid bumping it while entering or exiting a car.

* If you have more control, have your helper or family member grasp your unaffected upper arm at the elbow. Hold her elbow, and push down on your feet, until you can bounce yourself up to a standing position.

* If you use a walker or a cane, make sure they travel with you wherever you go.

4. Tips for Airline Travel

* Pack only what is necessary, and make sure you keep your medications with you at all times. Bring lightweight carry-on luggage that has wheels and a sturdy pull handle. Check with airline companies to make sure of regulations about carry-on luggage. A large canvas bag can hold your purse or other essential material. Tuck the bag under the seat in front of you and, if you need to use the overhead compartments, ask for assistance with lifting. It may be easier to check your luggage and bring one large carry-on bag with you. It may take more time to retrieve your luggage at your end destination, but you will not have to pull the luggage through huge airports.

* When making airline reservations, tell the airline representative that you have a disability and request a forward aisle seat on the airplane. Make sure you get a seat with a tray table that drops down from the seat ahead of you and not the kind that slides out from the armrest. The latter type of tray is too difficult to maneuver in cramped areas. Choose an aisle seat so that your affected side is toward the window in the row.

This protects your affected side from being bumped by other passengers, aids in easier access to the toilet, and aids in seeing around the airline cabin.

* Make arrangements ahead of time for any special mobility requests needed at your destination point and at airports where you are required to change planes. If you are not traveling in a wheelchair, a cart and driver can meet you and take you to your next destination. If you are in a wheelchair, an airline assistant can take you to your next plane or destination within the airport.

* If you are traveling in a wheelchair, keep the chair with you until you can transfer to the airline seat. It will be safely stored on the flight by the flight attendant until it is needed.

* All airline passengers with disabilities are allowed and encouraged to board the aircraft prior to standard passenger boarding.

* Remember to use the bathroom prior to boarding, because it may be difficult for you to use the airline toilet, especially in turbulent weather.

* If you do need to use the restroom, make sure you hold onto the grab bars located within each restroom. Take some toilet paper before sitting down so you will be able to find it more conveniently. Bring some disposable moist wipes or instant antibacterial hand-wash with you for easy clean up, because airliner faucets flow only when you push the handle. You can close the sink and fill a little water in the basin for easy hand washing as well.

* Ask the flight attendant for assistance when necessary.

* Buckle your seat belt by holding the insert portion close to your body with your affected hand for leverage and inserting the larger portion over it until it clicks. Pull snugly to secure.

5. Tips for Adaptive Recreation (gardening, bowling, golf, fishing, card games)

IT'S TIME TO PLAY. You deserve to find pleasure in those activities you enjoyed prior to your stroke. You've worked hard, and will continue to work within your recovery process, but now it's time to have fun. Almost all sports and recreational activities can be modified to support people with disabilities. The Courage Center is an excellent outlet for seasonal activities, indoor sports, and games as well (see the *Resource* section).

Adaptive Gardening

* Use adaptive equipment such as pulleys for hanging baskets and bird feeders.
* Use premade roll-out flowering strips that contain flower seeds instead of planting seeds individually.
* Modify garden design by raising flower beds to within easy reach and making garden paths wider.
* Growing things vertically may be easier than horizontally. Use a trellis or lattice type fencing to grow plants and flowers up.
* Wrap foam pipe insulation around hose nozzles or gardening tools for an easier grip.
* A small three-wheel pull cart is much better than a wheelbarrow. You can hang pockets on it to hold tools, too.
* Use Styrofoam™ packing balls or Styrofoam™ peanuts in the bottom of planters for proper drainage. They're lightweight and work great.
* Use a paste of flour and water to stick seeds on a strip of newspaper, then plant the entire strip. It's biodegradable.
* Use a soaker hose or sprinkler for watering versus holding the hose.
* A self-rewind hose is very useful.

Adaptive Bowling

* Most bowling centers have adaptable equipment available for bowlers. You can use a lightweight aluminum frame with a ramp that allows you to roll the ball down the ramp and toward the pins without having to lift the weight of the ball.
* Management can place inflatable devices in bowling alley

gutters to facilitate hitting the pins.

* Rather than wear bowling shoes, ask if the bowling center management will allow you to wear surgical booties over your street shoes, especially if you wear a brace. Surgical booties can be obtained at any hospital or hospital supply store.
* If you can't wear surgical booties over your street shoes, request two sizes of bowling shoes; one for your unaffected foot and a larger size to accommodate the brace on your affected foot.
* Seek assistance to step up onto the bowling floor and when handling the bowling ball.

Adaptive Golf

* Use a golf cart to facilitate walking long distances.
* Use bright-colored balls or balls that have beeper devices to aid in finding them.
* Grip the club and swing by leading with your unaffected hand and arm. Use a modified swing to improve accuracy.
* Practice at driving ranges and miniature golf courses to improve your swing and putting abilities.
* Golf small courses, and start with three holes instead of nine.
* Modify the clubs for your ability.
* Practice your swing without a ball in a large open space until you feel comfortable with the clubs again.
* Adaptive clubs are available, as well as Velcro™ fastened gloves, for improving support while gripping clubs.

Adaptive Fishing

* When in a boat, always wear a flotation device.
* If you are fishing from a small fishing boat, get into the boat from a dock by sitting on the dock, placing your feet in the boat, and sliding from the dock to the middle seat of the boat. Make sure you have assistance, because boats are extremely wobbly.
* Use a bright-colored bobber to alert you if a fish bites.
* Use live bait like worms, night crawlers, or minnows that can

be affixed to a larger hook using your unaffected hand.

* Use simple fishing poles, and fish from the shoreline.
* A harness device can be made or purchased that will hold your fishing pole against your body so that you can manipulate the reel with one hand.
* Most states offer free permanent fishing licenses for disabled individuals. Check with your state fish and wildlife licensing agency.

Adaptive Card Playing

* A block of wood with a groove cut in the middle and finely sanded to prevent splinters can be used to hold your hand of cards. Or, purchase plastic molded cardholders (see Figure 17).

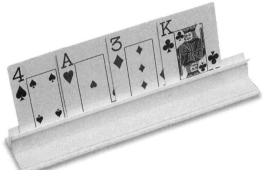

Figure 17. A plastic playing card holder.

Use an automatic shuffler for cards, so that you won't miss your turn at dealing. These shufflers can be obtained through catalogs offering recreational adaptability devices.

* To deal cards, splay them on the table in front of you so that they are all in your visual field. Use your unaffected fingers or thumb to count the cards and slide them to other players. Don't forget the player sitting on your affected side!
* Use a larger deck of cards to help you see the numbers and suits.
* Be patient with your ability. Games are supposed to be fun.
* Play simple games at first, and advance to more difficult games as your memory and tactile skills improve.

- Play solitaire on a computer. It lets you easily manipulate the cards as you relearn suits and numbers again.
- Computer card games are easier to play because you use a mouse, rather than handle actual cards. However, computer games also can lead to isolation. Use them sparingly. Socialization is a key factor in recreation and stroke recovery.

6. Tips for Driving Post-Stroke

WHEN WILL I be able to drive again? This question is best discussed by you, your neurologist, and the motor vehicle licensing office. Much of our independence hinges upon our ability to operate a motor vehicle, although we must be aware that driving is a privilege and not a right of citizenship. Your physician will determine when and if it is practical and advisable for you to get behind the wheel again. Stroke affects every individual differently, depending on what area of the brain is affected. When it comes to driving, safety must be paramount.

Because the ability to drive again can be a large issue in your progress towards independence, the following are some critical issues concerning stroke and driving, the proper procedure for checking your ability to drive after stroke, and general tips for driving.

Critical Issues

- Driving is the most serious accomplishment post-stroke, and the most dangerous.
- Driving should never be attempted post-stroke without the full consent of your neurologist, an accepted driving retraining course, and the motor vehicle licensing bureau.
- Some medications may impair your ability to safely operate a vehicle.
- A driver must be seizure free for at least 6 months before operating a motor vehicle. This requirement varies by state; check with your local DMV.
- Automobile insurance companies may decline your policy without proof or verification of a driving assessment certifi-

cate post-stroke. Don't drive without adequate auto insurance.

* Your car may have to be adapted to compensate for your stroke deficits. A driver's assessment program will instruct you regarding what type of equipment is best for you and your vehicle. Your car manufacturer or dealership also may be able to secure needed modifications and install them properly on your vehicle.

* An automatic transmission is easier to manipulate than a standard transmission for most people.

* Impaired cognition (the time it takes for the brain to process information) may reduce your reaction time.

* Your entire attention must be focused on driving. You must steer, watch your speed, watch for other cars and pedestrians, drive carefully, observe cars around you, follow traffic rules, and remember directions all at the same time.

* The ability to quickly process information, make prompt correct choices, follow directions, concentrate, understand cardinal points (north, south, east, and west), and see and hear what is happening around you is vitally important when driving.

* Your peripheral vision may be affected from stroke, or you may have other visual difficulties caused by stroke.

* Turn your head frequently while driving and practice visual scanning techniques to improve your field of view. Look ahead and focus on your path of travel, but at the same time, move your eyes and head right and left to notice what is occurring around you. Use your rear view mirror and side mirrors to see what is behind your vehicle.

* You may tire easily when driving. Rest frequently. Pull off the road into safe, well-lit rest areas when necessary.

* Driving depends on where you live. If you live in an area that has heavily congested traffic every day, consider hiring a car service or opting for other choices like public transportation or taxi service.

* You might be able to drive, but in the process, you may forget the big picture of where you're going. This is normal for some stroke heroes.

- Avoid unfamiliar areas until you feel confident about your driving ability.
- Plan your driving trips in advance by securing a large-print directional map that shows the route from departure to arrival address. Computer Web sites provide this service: www.MapQuest.com is one. Study the map before you start out, until you are certain that you understand each direction. If you get lost, pull over into a safe area and review the map.

Procedure for Driving after Stroke

After stroke, I was able to keep my driver's license for identification purposes, but with the understanding that I would not drive without permission from my neurologist. I waited 7 years before I felt medically stable and recovered enough to approach my neurologist on this issue.

- Take a course for rehabilitation and driver's safety through the Courage Center Driving Assessment Program. Payment for this course is offered at a sliding fee for qualified recipients. A driver's assessment program tests in a rehabilitation center vision, dexterity, recognition of roadway and pedestrian signs, as well as depth perception and other mandatory driving abilities. Once the assessment is made, you have the opportunity to get behind the wheel for a driver's training course. If and when you pass the test, you will receive a certificate stating you took the course.
- After renewing your license, and before driving again, have another vision test at the local motor vehicle licensing office.

Today, 12 years post-stroke, I continue to impose limits on myself for driving. I realize that the particular stroke I had affects my attention span; therefore, I do not drive when I am tired. I realize that my left peripheral vision is permanently affected by the stroke, and I compensate by turning my head to see traffic on my affected side. I realize that I cannot listen to the radio or a passenger's conversation and drive at the same time, so it must be quiet in the car at all times. My brain must be entirely focused on driving. I realize that unfamiliar and congested traffic areas may be beyond my driving ability, and I avoid them. I purchased a car that allowed me to install adaptability features for safety when driving. My driving is self-restricted by these essential safety guidelines.

General Tips for Driving

* Never use a cell phone while driving. Turn your cell phone off while driving; otherwise you could become startled or interrupted while concentrating on driving.
* Because of the increased number of accidents caused by cell phone use, such use while driving may be illegal in many areas, unless you have a hands-free phone system. But even a hands-free cell phone system may be too distracting for those of us with stroke difficulties.
* However, a cell phone is an extremely useful tool in case you have car trouble. Make sure you are parked in a safe area before using it. Keep the telephone number of emergency road service in your car. Many newer cars have an optional On Star® system for driving safety.
* Make sure your vehicle receives regular, proper maintenance.
* Good vision, and the ability to react to what you see, is crucial for safe driving.
* Glare caused by the sun, headlights, streetlights, and other light sources may inhibit vision in older drivers. This is due to physical changes within the eye that usually appear after age 50. Visit your eye doctor regularly.
* Wear your vehicle safety belt at all times while driving or as a passenger.
* Most states offer Driver Improvement Programs for people 55 years old and older. These 8-hour courses offer a 10 percent discount on most auto insurance and must be refreshed with a 4-hour course every 3 years. Check with your state department of public safety for details.

Brain Builders

1. Tips Regarding Relaxation

IT IS EXTREMELY important to rest often and even take a short nap every day. Your brain is healing, and you will find that your energy level and thinking skills wane if you push yourself to exhaustion. Your body will not permit long periods without rest. Your goal is to build new connections within the brain, and you must focus on allowing your body to rest and rejuvenate between periods of activity.

During my stroke recovery, I found the three M's to be very useful tools: *Mirrors, music,* and *meditation* were part of my home therapy routine. You may not find them listed in other stroke recovery books, but it certainly will not hurt you to add them as additional weapons within your arsenal of recovery. Mirrors and music will help you reassimilate the world around you; meditation may help in pain and stress relief.

* Mirrors are a very important piece of equipment in your process of recovery. Have several sizes, including a full-length mirror, at your disposal. Look into the bathroom mirror. While keeping your head stationary, look to the left. What do you see? Look to the right. What is reflected in the mirror? Can you name the things you saw while looking straight ahead?
* Now it's time for facial exercises. Smile as broadly as you can. Pucker your lips as if you are going to kiss someone. Stick your tongue out and move it slowly to the right and left. Close

one eye, then the other. Put your lips together as if you are blotting your lips. Open your mouth as far as possible and then close it. Blow to make your lips flutter. Move your tongue and pouch out one side of your mouth and then the other. Raise one eyebrow and then the other. Slowly try to make individual vowel sounds. Try saying simple words or your name. All these facial exercises are meant to stimulate the development of new brain activity and assist you in reclaiming your vital personality that shows through your face. I practice this technique daily and, over time, it helps me with applying makeup, learning to smile again, learning to move my eyes and head to see missed objects, and improving my self-esteem. Mirrors help me to realize that indeed I am a whole person. We are truly beautiful people.

* Music is an adaptive aid that has received little attention in formal therapy, but I have found it to be profoundly useful. I have several tapes and compact discs of soothing melodies that I use for relaxation, to help me sleep, and to relieve stress. While in the hospital, I used a tape recorder to play my favorite music to channel my thoughts into the music, instead of racing my brain on overdrive about things I could not control. Music continues to be an integral part of my life. When I listen to music, I focus on the sound. I listen and concentrate on the instruments' crescendos and tempo. Often, I fall asleep to the tune of a soft piano melody, knowing nothing I may be anxious about will change during the night. Tomorrow I will try again.

2. Tips for Alleviating Pain

A STRANGE PHENOMENON exists in our brain. Stroke, at least the ischemic type, does not cause pain, which is one reason why stroke warning signs may go unheeded. Pain usually brings us to the emergency room. Most stroke symptoms are painless and last only a few minutes, but can be deadly if not treated immediately. Our brain does not feel pain, yet we feel a headache. Migraines are not stroke symptoms. Stroke usually affects one side of the body. If stroke affects the thalamic region in our brain, we may experience sensations on the affected side of the body called central nerve pain or thalamic pain. For me, this pain is a constant tingling or icy feeling through my entire affected side, yet I cannot feel textures, water, hot or cold, or scratches, bumps, cuts, or bruises on this side of my body. This phenomenon is caused by incomplete or defective messages that are being sent from the brain to the affected side. If you have this condition, your neurologist may prescribe medication to help manage the discomfort. I choose to use meditation, relaxation techniques, and rest when I experience extreme thalamic pain, as I realize my brain is overworked and tired.

* Meditation or relaxation exercises play a large part in stroke recovery. Meditation is a form of *biofeedback*. Make sure you have a quiet place with no distractions prior to beginning this exercise. Here's how it works: While resting in bed or relaxing in a chair with your feet up, close your eyes and concentrate on the very top of your head. Relax your scalp. Relax the hair follicles that grow from your scalp. Working down, relax your forehead; all the worry lines seem to melt away. Relax your nose and upper cheeks. Now, relax the muscles of your chin, mouth, jaw, and lips. Work down your body, slowly naming the body part and concentrating on relaxing that particular part until you reach your toes. Don't forget the affected side of your body, even if you cannot feel it relaxing. Relax your shoulders and start with each side separately. Take your time with each body part before progressing to the next. Relax so that you can feel the soft heartbeat of your body pumping rhythmically. Breathe normally, pulling air in through your nostrils and out again. Picture in your mind the blood, rich in nutrients, flowing from your heart to your brain. Picture the brain using the fluid to nourish new areas. Picture the electrical impulses constantly humming within this marvelous human being. Think of your brain healing and nurturing your body. Over the 12 years that I have prac-

ticed this exercise, I can now easily meditate to ease aching muscles and relieve stress, and often I can avoid taking medication for pain. Meditation assists me with the central pain caused by the stroke affecting my thalamus. Pain medication makes me drowsy when I want to be alert. Central nervous pain is always a part of me. Meditation is how I deal with it on a daily basis.

3. Tips for Building New Connections within the Brain—Sensory Input

AFTER A STROKE, I found it very difficult to position myself into a comfortable position in bed, because my stroke-affected side would no longer move to my command. Within a few months, I could flop over onto my affected side, but found it difficult to move back. I felt as if I was falling. I quickly learned that:

* A large body pillow stationed against my back with a smaller pillow between my knees alleviated this problem.
* To improve sensory input, I would lie on my affected side for a very short period every night and roll onto my back for relief. Central nerve pain has plagued me since the stroke, and this exercise seemed to exacerbate it during the first few months. But by lengthening the time spent lying on my affected side, I have increased the amount of tolerance between my brain and the affected area. I began to feel new sensations throughout affected body parts. Over time, my body has adjusted, and I do not feel as if I am going to fall when lying on my affected side. Although I continue to be unaware of my affected side when the bedroom light is off, I can move my body into a comfortable sleeping position and shift the affected side more smoothly.
* You may find that you want to protect your stroke-affected side by holding your affected arm with your unaffected hand. This is good for sensory input. But take it a step further and touch every part of your affected side. Knead your affected

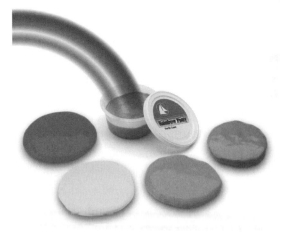

Figure 18. Pressure-sensitive putty is used for hand exercises.

fingers and hand with your unaffected hand when you're watching television or relaxing in a chair. If you wear a brace on your affected arm, feel your affected fingers and try to bend them or wiggle them with your unaffected fingers. Try to move your affected fingers on their own. Even if your affected fingers move a fraction of an inch, that's progress.

* Touching material of various textures with your affected hand stimulates affected areas in your brain. Lace your unaffected fingers between your affected fingers and place the palm and fingers of your affected hand on various fabrics and surfaces. This may feel very strange at first, but you are rewiring brain pathways as well as becoming aware of spatial fields on your affected side.

* Figure 18 shows a material called Rainbow Putty, which indicates by color the resistance of the material to your grip.

* Use a hand exerciser to improve sensation and strength in your affected hand. The Thera-Band® Hand Exerciser is shown in Figure 19.

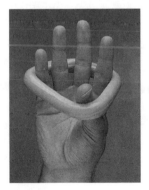

Figure 19. A hand exerciser.

Aromatherapy is a great way to recondition your sense of smell while you relax. Here are some ideas to assist sensory input in this area.

* Purchase a small compact disc player that offers different scents on assorted CDs.
* Use scented oils in a potpourri pot.
* Simmer in a small amount of water the herbs and flavorings found in your spice rack, like cinnamon sticks, lemon, or vanilla. These scents enhance your sense of well-being.
* I strongly advise against using candles as a form of aromatherapy when at home, unless you are with another adult who assumes the responsibility of designated candle-snuffer.

4. Tips for Organization

As Jonathan Winters said in the movie, *The Russians Are Coming*, "We've got to get organized!"

Organization assists our minds in healing. Disarray bombards our senses with overstimulation.

* Keep a journal of your progress and add important information such as medications and doctors' phone numbers to the notebook too.
* An accordion-type file works great for keeping hospital information, therapy center handouts, and information about stroke support groups.
* A different color accordion file can hold medical bills in order of provider.
* Keep a communication board or letter board at ready access if you are having aphasic difficulties.
* You may find it useful to keep a small tape recorder and cassette tape ready, because it is useful for giving short, direct instructions and reminders. Also, with the permission of others, use it to tape conversations for recall when short-term memory is affected.
* Opening your mail can be accomplished by using a letter opener and stabilizing the letter with your affected elbow or grasping it between your knees. If you cannot grasp the letter in this manner, place the bottom of the letter in a top

drawer, close the drawer so that the letter is sticking out, and use the letter opener with your unaffected hand.

* To mail a letter in a mailbox, put the letter on top of the mailbox, or if weather is the weather is bad, hold the letter between your pursed lips or under your affected arm while you open the mailbox. Place your unaffected elbow on the lid to hold it down, and use your unaffected hand to grab the letter and drop it inside the box. Move your unaffected elbow out of the lid by moving your arm down to catch the lid with your hand and fingers. Use your fingers to let go of the mailbox lid. Another way is to quickly pull your elbow up out of the way of the lid.

* To fold letters for mailing, stabilize the top of the letter with a book or another handy, heavy object so it won't slide away. With the palm of your hand, roll the bottom one third of the way up. Crease it with the palm of your hand and finish creasing with your fingers. Turn the letter around and do the same procedure to the other side so that it is folded in thirds. Hold the envelope with the open flap toward you between your knees or stabilize it with your affected forearm. Stuff the envelope, wet it lightly with a damp sponge, and close it. Use the self-adhesive type of postage stamps that peel off their backings like stickers and plop one on.

5. Tips for Exercising the Stroke-Affected Side of Your Body

IF NEW THE CONNECTIONS formed within the brain are not continuously stimulated, our affected side will get weaker and our unaffected side will become stronger. Formal therapy is our beginning point, but we must take the techniques learned in rehabilitation back home with us and continue to exercise our stroke-affected areas.

* Remember good posture. Sit up straight and arch your back every once in a while. Drop your shoulders and stretch your neck so that your head is perfectly erect.

- Try to put both feet together on the floor when sitting. Then, move one foot out a few inches and try to have the affected foot follow. Now try the opposite side. Don't hook your foot behind the other to move it, but see if you can slide it by moving your knee and lower leg.

- I practiced an old Laurel and Hardy comedy routine as part of my daily exercise to build eye–hand coordination, fine motor skills, speed, and dexterity during recovery. Pat your thighs, clap your hands, and reach for the ear opposite your affected hand and your nose with your unaffected hand. Your arms should cross at the wrist and forearm. Again, pat your thighs, clap your hands, and reach for your nose with your affected hand and reach for your opposite ear with your unaffected hand. Begin slowly and work to increase your speed over time. Try this exercise your eyes shut, then open.

- Stand with your affected shoulder against a wall. Spread your feet out for improved balance. Hold onto the back of a sturdy chair with your unaffected side, if necessary. If you are in a wheelchair, position the chair as close to the wall as possible and lock the brakes. Place your affected hand, palm spread if possible, on the wall. Use your fingers to slowly climb your hand up the wall as far as possible. Have a family member place a small pencil mark on the highest point you can reach. Each day, try to reach higher. Move very slowly at first, because this exercise can be difficult. If you have a *frozen shoulder*, a shoulder joint that does not move, formal therapy may be necessary before attempting this exercise.

- Touch and gently massage your affected side as much and as often as possible. This excites brain neurons to sensation and touch. This gentle effort can assist you in your awareness of your affected side and prevent neglect.

- Join a local hospital exercise class or call your local stroke support group to inquire about exercise classes for stroke survivors.

- The American Heart Association/American Stroke Association has an exercise videotape available for stroke survivors. (See the section on *Resources*.)

6. Tips for Television Program Viewing that Builds Brain Power

ALTHOUGH MANY MAY people say that being a couch potato is a bad thing, some television programs build and rebuild brainpower.

* Quiz shows that highlight multiple choice answers are best for playing along. *Jeopardy,* in which you must phrase your answer in the form of a question, may be more difficult. If you know the answer, try saying it aloud. Don't worry about forming a question. Try to say the first thing that pops into your mind. If you're involved in the program, you may not be as self-conscious about speech difficulties. Try to trick your brain into using other avenues for retrieving information. Increased automatic reflexes are part of the stroke recovery process.
* *Jeopardy, Who Wants to Be a Millionaire, Family Feud,* and other quiz shows, as well as the programming available on the Public Broadcasting Service (PBS), such as *NOVA,* will not magically turn you into a couch potato. Selective television viewing can, on the contrary, be beneficial toward rejuvenating brainpower.

Television viewing has another benefit for post-stroke that you may have never considered: Advertisers have about 30 seconds of air time to catch viewers' attention in selling their products. Because television advertisements usually occur rapidly and in succession, I have a difficult time remembering them. This results in poor product recognition and decreased spending.

* If you want to increase your brainpower, try to remember as many advertisements as you can between programming. Turn off the television after watching a few ads and try to recite the products being sold in as many advertisements as you can remember.
* The caveat to this exercise is that you may have difficulty remembering the original program you were viewing.

Perform either programming retention or advertisement retention by muting the sound.

7. Tips for Using a Computer

COMPUTER USERS SHOULD be aware of both the good and bad news associated with technology use. So, hang onto your mouse and don't press the Delete key until I explain.

* The good news is that whether you choose an IBM-compatible or Macintosh computer, your world will be open to an easier and faster way of doing many tasks.
* Software are the programs installed on your computer. These programs may allow you to do things more easily, like keeping track of your household budget or simply typing a letter and saving it for future reference. For a small additional monthly fee, a computer can allow you to surf the Web through access to the Internet.
* Hardware, such as computer screens and keyboards, can be enlarged or adapted to meet your needs.
* A computer can allow you to easily keep in touch with family and friends all over the world by accessing the Internet and e-mail.
* The Internet is usually accessible if you have a home computer, and it provides a wealth of information.
* Basic computer classes are available through community education classes, business schools, community colleges, and universities.
* Don't be afraid to play with your computer. Open a software program and experiment with the wonderful opportunities and choices it offers. The best way to learn is by doing.
* Voice recognition software allows the computer to type the words you say. A microphone headset is included in these software packages. It will take time to train the software to recognize your voice and correctly spell the words you say. But after you familiarize yourself with the program, it may

become a great tool for you.

* A calculator comes as part of standard software packages for computers. Many types of financial management software are available. Computer programs can keep track of vital financial information and, if you have provided the information, software programs can easily prepare your taxes.

* The bad news is that working at a computer is usually a solo activity, and it is easy to get so engrossed in doing an activity that you forget there is a real world around you to be explored.

* A computer needs maintenance and protection against viruses. By using the Internet, it is easy to open and download an unsuspected computer virus that has the potential of making your computer unusable. Don't download anything that is not reviewed by your virus protection software first, and only open e-mail or attachments if you know the sender.

8. Tips for a Home Office

IF YOU ARE ABLE to return to work, check with your employer to see if you can do your work from home and correspond via your home computer. This will not only save travel time, but conserve your energy as well. If you are not able to return to your employment, check with the Department of Vocational and Rehabilitation Services in your area for retraining opportunities.

A home office might be a great way for you to provide volunteer or paid employment. However, check with your neurologist first to find out what adaptive measures she recommends for your work routine. You may find that you tire easily, and your attention span may be limited. A home office provides for short periods of work and the opportunity for comfortable rest too. If you decide to implement a home office, I used the following tips to make work easier after my stroke:

* Designate a room on the main floor of your home for your office.

* Install a wide L-shaped desk with plenty of file cabinets and lots of open workspace.
* Place a desktop computer in the corner of the desk area.
* Use a comfortable high-back chair.
* Install mini blinds or other easy accessible window treatments that can be cleaned and operated with one hand.
* Organize office supplies on a turntable within close reach on your unaffected side.
* Have a cordless phone nearby, preferably one with a speakerphone and answering system built in.
* If you use the telephone frequently, use a headset on your telephone system.
* Type frequently used telephone numbers in a large bold font, print them, place the 8-?" by 11" sheet of paper in a picture frame, and hang it directly above your desktop phone.
* Use stackable bins on wheels to store frequently used paperwork.
* Use bookshelves to store reference material within easy reach.
* Make sure computer peripherals, such as printers and scanners, are within easy reach.
* Other items I have found useful are a tall coffee cup for holding pens, a cassette tape recorder with plenty of batteries and fresh tapes for that sudden burst of enlightenment, self-adhesive preaddressed labels, a Rolodex? for business cards, sticky notes, a cassette carousal for computer programs and recording tapes, a fan or central air conditioning, a paper shredder, and a utility drawer.

Here are some ideas for home office jobs you might consider post-stroke:

* Consultant
* Newsletter editor
* Travel agent
* Secretarial service
* Marketing and selling handmade items

* Freelance writing
* Business planner
* Web site design
* Web or Internet research
* Your expertise and combine it with a new idea for marketing
* be creative!

In addition to actually working over the Internet, many colleges and universities provide online courses so that you can earn a degree without leaving home.

9. Tips and Tidbits

LET'S SAY THAT you were invited to a birthday party at the White House. Yikes! You'll have to bring a present and wrap it too. Don't worry. Go to the nearest Dollar Store, buy a gift, and buy a gift bag and some fancy tissue paper too.

* Roll the gift in tissue, plop it in a bag, and place another piece of tissue in the bag so that the ends stick out.
* Another way to get a fancy gift wrapped is to have it gift wrapped at the store you purchase the gift from. It may cost a few dollars, but they do a professional job at wrapping, and you can choose the paper, bow, and gift card.

You just bought a CD of your favorite vocalist and can't open the hermetically sealed disc. Don't fret; you can do it.

* Place the CD in your kitchen cutting board vise grip. Use a sharp knife to cut the cellophane wrapping across one end and peel it off the rest of the CD. Placing it back in the vise, taped edge up, pry the knife tip under the tape until you can get hold of it to pull it off. Take the CD out of the gripper and lay it flat, with the opening to your unaffected side. Flip it open with your fingers.
* Or (and this is my all-time favorite), have a store clerk open

the CD for you at the time of purchase. Don't feel obligated to explain your disability; just ask the clerk to open it for you. They're difficult to open for everyone.

If you want to clip coupons out of the newspaper or magazine for your weekly shopping:

* Use an old card table or a wide empty counter top for a surface. Place a paperweight on the open newspaper to hold it in place. With the scissors slightly open, use the bottom edge of the scissors as forceps to pick up the outer edge of the coupon. Make sure you use your unaffected hand to cut out the coupon. Don't worry if you didn't do it perfectly the first time. This takes practice. The coupon will be accepted even if you cut a little wider than the dotted line indicated.

It's time to tear paper off a paper towel roll or toilet tissue roll. Here's how you can do it one-handed without getting the entire roll spinning out of control.

* Take the amount you need and then, with the index finger and thumb of your unaffected hand, break the first few perforations of the tissue. Place the back of your fingers against the roll for support and tear the rest off by using the same process, your thumb and index finger.

You want to hang clothes on a clothesline, but can't figure out how to do it without bending, stretching, and having the clothes fall off the line. Let's try an easy way.

* Get a hamper or wheeled cart to set your clothes basket on so that the basket is about waist level. Place the garment over the clean line. Put a clothespin on it to stabilize the item. Readjust the garment with one clothespin at a time then release the stabilizing clothespin.

10. Tips for Pet Owners after Stroke

OWNING A PET is a big responsibility. Animals need daily care too. They require food, fresh water, exercise, frequent veterinarian check-ups and immunizations, grooming, city licensing if necessary, and lots of love.

If you have a pet that has been with your family before your stroke, the animal may be a great comfort to you when you return from the hospital after your stroke. However, there are some issues of pet ownership that you should be aware of after a stroke.

- If you have a small dog or a cat, be aware that the animal may come up to you on your affected side, where you may not be able to see it. Be extremely careful that your pet does not trip you.
- Make sure your dog or cat is spayed or neutered.
- Make sure you know where your pet is before using a walker or cane to move about. Your new equipment may appear to be a plaything to your animal.
- If you have a bird, make sure the cage is cleaned daily and that the bird has fresh water and the proper type of birdseed. Some people cover the cage at night to quiet their bird for sleep.
- A well-filtered aquarium, large enough for the number of fish, and a small amount of fish food daily will adequately support the easy maintenance of fish.
- Your medical risk must be weighed carefully against the risk of owning an animal before getting a pet after your stroke. Will you be able to care for the pet properly? Will the pet interfere with your mobility? Will you be able to pet-proof your home? Does your apartment management accept pets? Who will care for the pet if you are away? Talk with a veterinarian about the care of a particular animal before you bring the new pet home.
- You are making, or have made, a major commitment to an animal, and the responsibility for his care is up to you and your family.

I had a small dog that was our family pet before and after my stroke. This miniature schnauzer would bark, run, jump, and get excited over the most unusual things. However, this dog would also not leave a bedside when someone was sick. It was as if the dog had taken on a role of "family protector." The family dog provided me with a great sense of love, familiarity, and belonging when I came home from the hospital after my stroke. Pets also provide you with someone to talk to when you are alone, even if they don't understand everything you say. Pets love attention, so go ahead and talk; they will respond to your voice inflection.

When I lived independently, I had a cockatiel bird. By teaching the bird to talk, I taught myself to talk as well?one word, or short phrase, repeated over and over again until the bird became accustomed to my tone of voice and was able to repeat the word. However, my cockatiel insisted on talking when I was on the telephone. Apparently, he thought I was talking to him and would screech and prattle until I covered the cage as a signal of quiet time. I owned Kato the cockatiel for 5 or 6 years, all through college. Unconsciously, I'd say, "Be quiet. I'm studying." And the bird would repeat my constant mantra. The cockatiel bird was a hilarious and somewhat easy pet to care for. I learned to clip wings and talons one-handed. I learned to use a T-bar as a safety perch when the bird flew to inaccessible areas. I learned to care for something other than myself, and this is marvelous therapy.

Now, I have a cat that I've had since he was a kitten. The veterinarian and I decided that the kitten be declawed because of my high risk for anticoagulant medications. This is a very volatile issue in cat ownership. In some countries, this procedure is considered illegal. Make sure you discuss this course of action with a well-qualified veterinarian and that your animal is at the proper age and health before arranging for this alteration. The kitten or cat should not be allowed outside once he has been declawed. Kittens and cats are instinctively curious. They will follow you and rub against your leg as a way of marking their owner. However, these natural cat responses could trip you if you are not careful. Learn your cats' usual behavior, and then be prepared for the unexpected. My cat is a lap cat. Buddy will jump onto my lap to be petted and brushed. I am prepared for this habit and enjoy his company. Sometimes, I place an old towel across my lap for him to lie on. This prevents the cat's shed fur from adhering to clothing. A pet hair remover brush, lint brush, and frequent vacuuming can also be used to prevent pet shedding and allergic reactions. Special pet shampoos may decrease reactions to pet allergies. By pouring the liquid onto a large sponge and wiping down the cat, the allergies caused by cat fur or dander are lessened. Buddy also wears a small bell on his collar that alerts me when he is near. My cat is never allowed in the kitchen when I am cooking or eating. Food is always stored properly to prevent the cat from investigating kitchen territory. I place a cat treat on the top step of the open basement stairway prior to preparing meals. Buddy goes for the treat, and I gently close the door. After meal-time and dishes are done, Buddy is allowed to come upstairs to join me. He quickly learned that treats are given for his good behavior. Buddy meow at the office door if I've been at the computer too long. He signals me that he wants attention. He is the management telling me it's break time.

SECTION VIII

The Importance of Love

LOVE BEGINS WITH a touch, a look, a hug, a smile, a thought, and a need for intimacy. Love is communication on a human level. Women may feel that they are not as appealing after their stroke as they were before. Men may experience erectile dysfunction. Some medications may have an effect on your libido.

- If the desire for sexual intercourse is intact, and not muted by some types of antidepressant medication, begin to verbalize your desire to your partner.
- Sometimes a stroke may mute the ability to read innuendoes. In this case, be specific in your communication about the desire to have intercourse. The most romantic, direct, and uplifting statement to make or to hear is, "I would like to make love with you."
- An open discussion with your physician may alleviate you and your partner's concerns about resuming sexual intercourse.
- You are the same person as before the stroke, even if you may be experiencing personality or physical differences post-stroke.
- Every person requires intimacy to some degree, and relationships begin in the heart.
- Reevaluate your marriage/partnership commitment. What specific adjectives describe your marriage or partnership? Life partner, sharing, love, parenting, pledge, vow, promise, sexuality, faithfulness, and unity, are all words that may be

used to describe your devotion to each other.

* Continue to enhance your unity in the face of adversity. Sometimes dedication is strengthened by difficulties as long as you continue to grow together.

1. Tips to Improve Intimacy

STROKE MAY CAUSE self-image difficulties for some people. Help them to understand that you still love them.

* If you, as a partner, are experiencing emotional problems toward resuming sexual relations with your stroke hero, consult professional counseling.
* Thrive on love. Make time for your partner and grow together, not apart.
* Stop labeling. You are husband, wife, or lover before you are caregiver or stroke survivor.
* Sexuality begins in the brain. How you use what you have can make for a very satisfying sexual experience.
* Your partner will enjoy the experience more knowing that you possess a unique creative flair.
* Many people who have had a stroke go on to lead a very satisfactory sex life.
* Have fun and enjoy yourself and your partner.
* Share your fantasies. Everyone has them!
* Your sexual experience is unique to your mind and body experience. Sexual intercourse is part of our human desires. If libido is affected by the stroke, it may take time before the desire for a sexual experience returns. Talk openly with your partner about sexual issues. Consult your neurologist for explanations when necessary.
* A sex therapist (yes, there are such specialties) may be helpful in explaining how you and your partner can satisfy your mutual needs.
* Consult your physician for medication for erectile dysfunction. Be aware that other medications you may be taking for

blood pressure or other conditions may cause contraindications.

* Use a latex condom to avoid sexually transmitted diseases (STDs) and autoimmune deficiency (HIV/AIDS). Stroke does not mean that we can forget that there are diseases out there. Protect yourself and your loved one. Practice safe sex.

2. Tips for Positioning

* Communicate to your partner what position is the most appropriate for relaxation, touch, and movement.
* You will not have another stroke because of sexual intercourse.
* Try various forms of sexual activity for arousal such as extended foreplay or oral stimulation.
* Lie on your unaffected side or back for better control and balance.

3. Tips for Touch and Sight

* Keep the lights on. You may not be aware of your stroke-affected side if you can't see it. Visual stimulation may be improved as well.
* Communicate to your partner exactly what part of your body has been affected by the stroke and request manipulation of the unaffected side.
* Remember that partners are not mind readers. If you are having difficulty communicating because of the stroke, use hand movements and facial expressions to indicate pleasurable touch.

Families Need Care Too

1. Tips for Family Members

STROKE AFFECTS FAMILY relationships too. The indirect repercussions of stroke will affect each family member. Psychologists, neurologists, and medical staff associated with stroke centers and rehabilitation facilities all agree that stroke has a profound affect on family dynamics. Everyone needs to feel loved. Not only will it be your responsibility to assist your loved one during stroke recovery, but you will be the one to carry on the normal daily routines as well. If you are employed, any dreams of early retirement may have vanished. While your stroke hero is working at improving, you may be faced with the responsibility of handling family finances, shopping, childcare if children are in the home, cooking, cleaning, laundry, and home maintenance. This stressful situation is even further complicated by your concern for the health and welfare of your loved one. In time, your loved one may improve. Time becomes a four-letter word in stroke recovery. But time may become your ally too.

* Take time to evaluate your family dynamics. Over the course of time, how does your relationship change? Usually, our lives get busier, and we tend to take things for granted. This is normal and natural.
* Reflection exercise: Review your family dynamics before the

stroke. On half of a sheet of paper write down what your family did regularly before the stroke. What were your children doing? What was the picture of your family? How did you feel about each other? Where were you financially? Were both partners working full-time or part-time? Who was mainly responsible for what tasks? Name specific tasks and who preformed them on a regular basis.

In another column, jot down words that explain how the stroke changed your life. Examples are fear, nursing duties, stress, financial vulnerability, and unknown future. Underneath, write how you think the stroke affected your loved one. Examples may be immediate loss of power and control, alteration to family structure, loss of independence, communication difficulties, financial hardships, intimacy, depression, resentment, frustration, negativity, and stress on the relationship. On another sheet of paper, number the ways that you can handle each situation in a positive way. You have now opened the channels of communication by working together. You have concretely written all, or most, negativity down. Keep only the positive steps and try, each day, to work towards them.

Your family dynamics and marriage have changed. Some changes came over the course of time, and others because of the stroke. No one understands how much stroke has affected your life as well as you and your partner. All marriages take work to stay strong. Communicate effectively. In time, ease back on taking everything as your personal responsibility. Give as much responsibility, power, and freedom to your partner as is safely possible. They may surprise you.

* Join a stroke caregiver support group through your local hospital or rehabilitation facility.
* Plan time for yourself at least once a week. An evening out with friends or even a weekend away can be a terrific stress reliever.
* Exercise daily. Walk around the block or join a class with friends.

* Make time for your hobbies and interests, because they are vitally important too.
* Call on friends, neighbors, relatives, coworkers, or church members to visit and assist you with care once in a while. Company will help both of you to feel less isolated and alone. Additional help will be a welcomed attribute.
* Empathy is good, but sympathy is poison to your stroke hero. They're relying on you to understand and encourage them every step of the way.
* When you visit the doctor with your stroke hero, bring written questions along that apply to you too. Caring for someone who has had a stroke is an awesome responsibility, and you will need help through this journey of recovery.
* Most important, ask the neurologist to show you the MRI of your stroke hero and explain the areas affected by the stroke and the functions of each affected area. Empowering you with knowledge will make you better prepared for adaptable techniques.

2. Positive Strokes

* Assist in giving responsibility back to your partner. First, this act of sharing duties takes the burden from other family members. Second, it provides for independence. Finally, it is a positive way to heal.
* At least once a week, allow your partner to be responsible for some type of meal planning, cooking, cleaning, bill paying, laundry, parenting decisions, and family management responsibilities. Stroke heroes need to be a necessary part of the family again.
* You are not responsible for your partner's feelings.
* Use parroting techniques to assist communication. Examples of parroting statements are, "I hear you saying…" or, "It hurts me when you said…." Repeat the words you heard your partner say. This method clarifies statements said and heard, opens the door for direct messages to be interpreted and com-

municated, and avoids frustration.

* Family members should avoid saying things like, "Do this because it will be good therapy." Stroke heroes are no longer in therapy, but are trying to live life to the best of their capabilities and learn new ways of adapting to their environment.

3. Tips about Children

CHILDREN HAVE STROKES TOO. But we address here the reaction of young family members, especially preschoolers, to a parent or grandparent who has had a stroke. Little ones depend on adults for so many things. Too often, they are forgotten about in the healing process, because so much attention is focused on the patient and the caregiver. Children might regress to bedwetting, daytime diapers, baby talk, whining, or other negative behavior. This is a normal reaction to a traumatic event in their lives. Preschoolers keenly sense stressful situations, even if they don't understand the problem.

* Spend time with your child on a one-to-one basis.
* Crouch down to your child's level and address the child face–to-face over important matters.
* Explain what has happened in terms your child understands.
* Give your child very simple tasks to do, like folding wash-cloths or matching socks, so that little helpers feel part of the healing process.
* Make a simple chart for them, and place stickers or stars on it for daily positive behavior and accomplished tasks. When they earn a certain number of stickers, they win a new book, for example. Avoid giving food, candy, or expensive toys as a reward.
* Have young children help in the care of your stroke hero as much as safety allows. They can play with the Thera-Putty™ too. They can share a picture book. They can help set the table or pick up their toys so that no one trips on small objects.
* Children have a terrific capacity of adaptability. Maybe your

little ones can create new approaches to performing a task for you.

* Answer their questions honestly. If you don't know the answer, tell them that too! But tell them that you are working together every day at getting better. Children need hope. Children need to know that you will be there for them.

SECTION X

Help is
On the Way

IT IS IMPORTANT to know that you and your family are not alone. According to the American Stroke Association and National Stroke Association 2004 statistics, on average, someone suffers a stroke every 45 seconds. About 750,000 Americans suffer strokes each year. Every 3.3 minutes, someone dies of a stroke. Today, there are 4.7 million stroke survivors, and this figure is expected to rise as the Baby Boom generation continues to age and medical and stroke rehabilitation accelerates. The annual cost of stroke in the United States is $55 billion in lost wages and medical care, and this figure will also climb with our aging population. Stroke is the leading diagnosis from hospital to long-term care. These statistics are cited to let you know that you are not alone, and that agencies, medical personnel, and community resources are available to assist you and your family.

* Reach out to available resources for assistance for your particular needs.

Resources (in alphabetical order)

1. Adaptive Gardening Tools and Equipment

A.M. Leonard, Inc.
241 Fox Drive
Piqua, OH 45356-0816
1-800-433-0633
www.amleo.com

Charley's Greenhouse & Garden
17979 State Rt. 536 (Memorial Hwy.)
Mount Vernon, WA
1-800-322-4707, ext. 3001
www.charleysgreenhouse.com

Gardener's Supply Company
128 Intervale Road
Burlington, VT 05401
1-888-833-1412
www.gardeners.com

Smith & Hawken, Ltd.
P.O. Box 8690
Pueblo, CO 81008-9998
1-800-940-1170
www.smithandhawken.com

Lee Valley Tools, Ltd.
P.O. Box 1780
Ogdensburg, NY 13669-6780
1-800-871-8158 USA
1-800-267-8767 Canada
www.leevalley.com

2. Associations and Organizations

American Association of Retired Persons (AARP)
601 E Street NW
Washington, DC 20049
1-800-424-2277
www.aarp.org

ACTION
1100 Vermont Avenue NW
Washington, DC 20525
202-606-4855 (Call for number of regional office.)
This federal agency sponsors older American volunteer programs that include Retired Senior Volunteer Program (RSVP) and Senior Companion Program, in which volunteers provide assistance so that low-income people age 60 and over can remain in their homes.

American Academy of Neurology
1080 Montreal Avenue
St. Paul, MN 55116-2311
651-695-2791
www.aan.com

American Dietetic Association/National Center for Nutrition and Dietetics
216 West Jackson Boulevard
Chicago, IL 60606-6995
1-800-366-1655 (Consumer Nutrition Hotline)
www.eatright.org
Consumers may speak to a registered dietitian for answers to nutrition questions or obtain a referral to a local registered dietitian.

American Health Assistance Foundation
22512 Gateway Center Drive
Clarksburg, MD 20871
Tel: 301-948-3244 or 1-800-437-AHAF (2423)
Fax: 301-258-9454
info@ahaf.org
www.ahaf.org

American Heart Association/American Stroke Association
7272 Greenville Avenue
Dallas, TX 75231-4596
1-888-4-STROKE (1-888-478-7653)
www.strokeassociation.org

American Stroke Association
1-800-553-6321
Information and referral service offering free stroke support
information to stroke survivors, family members, caregivers,
and health professionals.

American Speech-Language-Hearing Association
10801 Rockville Pike
Rockville, MD 20852
1-800-638-8255
www.asha.org

Brain Aneurysm Foundation
12 Clarendon Street
Boston, MA 02116
Tel: 617-723-3870
Fax: 617-723-8672
information@bafound.org
www.bafound.org

Bungalow Software, Inc.
2905 Wakefield Drive
Blacksburg, VA 24060-8184
1-800-891-9937
www.bungalowsoftware.com
Bungalow offers computer software to assist in recovering speech
and language after stroke.

Children's Hemiplegia and Stroke Association (CHASA)
4101 West Green Oaks Blvd.
PMB #149
Arlington, TX 76016
817-492-4325
info5@chasa.org
www.hemikids.org

Courage Center
3915 Golden Valley Road
Golden Valley, MN 55422-9984
763-588-0811 or 1-888-846-8253
www.courage.org

Medicare Hotline
1-800-MEDICARE (1-800-633-4227)

Mobility International
P.O. Box 10767
Eugene, OR 97440
541-343-1284

National Aphasia Association
29 John Street, Suite 1103
New York, NY 10038
1-800-922-4622
www.aphasia.org

National Easter Seal Society
230 West Monroe Street, Suite 1800
Chicago, IL 60606
312-726-6200 (or check telephone book for local Easter Seal Society)
This organization provides information and services to help people with many disabilities, including those caused by stroke. Rehabilitation services include physical, occupational, and speech therapy as well as vocational evaluation, training, and placement.

National Institute of Neurological Disorders and Stroke
(NINDS)
P.O. Box 5801
Bethesda, MD 20824
1-800-352-9424
www.ninds.nih.gov

National Stroke Association
9707 East Easter Lane
Englewood, CO 80112
1-800-STROKES (1-800-787-6537)
www.stroke.org

North Coast Medical, Inc.
18305 Sutter Boulevard
Morgan Hill, CA 95037-2845
Their catalog, Functional Solutions, can be ordered by calling
1-800-235-7054.
www.BeAbleToDo.com

Peterson Press
Stroke Awareness and Recovery
121 West Saint Marie Street
Duluth, MN 55803-2613
218-728-5788

Residential Aphasia Program
Communicative Disorders Clinic
University of Michigan
1111 East Catherine Street
Ann Arbor, MI 48109-2054
313-764-8440

Social Security Administration
Office of Public Inquiries
Windsor Park Building
6401 Security Boulevard
Baltimore, MD 21235
1-800-772-1213
www.socialsecurity.gov

Stroke Clubs International
805 12th Street
Galveston, TX 77550
409-762-1022
Stroke survivors operate this organization. They promote the hiring of people with disabilities and provide lists of stroke clubs in each state.

Telephone Equipment Distribution Program
www.TEDPA.org
www.TedProgram.org
These programs offer state programs, either income or needs-based, for TTY services, CAPTEL, Speak Easy, speakerphones, or picture phones.

The Department of Vocational/Rehabilitation Services
Find local listings in your telephone book's Government section.
www.ssa.gov

The National Library Service for the Blind and Physically Handicapped (NLS)
Library of Congress
Washington, DC 20542
Mailing Address: 1291 Taylor Street NW
Washington, DC 20011
1-800-424-8567
www.loc.gov/nls

The Stroke Network
A Web-based stroke support and referral organization.
www.strokenetwork.org

The Well Spouse Foundation
P.O. Box 801
New York, NY 10023
1-800-838-0879
Provides support for husbands, wives, and partners of people
who are chronically ill or disabled.

3. Books (Additional Readings):

Breslin, Jimmy. I Want to Thank My Brain for Remembering
Me. Boston: Little Brown & Co., 1996.

Burkman, Kip. The Stroke Recovery Book: A Guide for Patients
and Families. Omaha: Addicus Books, Inc.,1998.

Caplan, Louis MD, Dyken, Mark MD, and Easton, J. Donald MD.
American Heart Association Family Guide to Stroke Treatment,
Recovery, and Prevention. New York: Times Books, 1996.

Donahue, Peggy Jo. How to Prevent a Stroke: A Complete Risk
Reduction Program. Emmaus, PA: Rodale Press, 1989.

Donnan, Geoffrey M.D., and Burton, Carol. After a Stroke: A
Support Book for Patients, Caregivers, Families, and Friends.
Berkley, CA: North Atlantic Books, 1990.

Haggard, Jerry W. I Had a Stroke and Survived. Salt Lake City,
UT: Northwest Publishing, 1994.

Hutton, Cleo, and Caplan, Louis R. MD. Striking Back at Stroke:
A Doctor-Patient Journal. New York: Dana Press, 2003.

Klein, Bonnie Sherr. Out of the Blue: One Woman's Story of Stroke, Love, and Survival. Berkley, CA: Wildcat Canyon Press and Persimmon Blackbridge, 1998.

Larkin, Marilynn, and Sonberg, Lynn. When Someone You Love has a Stroke. New York: Dell Publishing Co., 1995.

McCrum, Robert. My Year off Recovering Life after a Stroke. New York: W.W. Norton, 1998.

Mayer, Tommye-Karen. One Handed in a Two-Handed World. Boston: Prince Gallison Press, 1996.

Restak, Richard. The Secret Life of the Brain. New York: Dana Press and Joseph Henry Press, 2001.

Sacks, Oliver. The Man Who Mistook His Wife for a Hat: And Other Clinical Tales. New York: Harper & Row, 1987.

Sarino, John E., and Martha Taylor Sarino. Stroke: The Condition and the Patient. New York: McGraw-Hill, 1969.

Swaffield, Laura. Stroke: The Complete Guide to Recovery and Rehabilitation. Northamptonshire, England: Thorsons Publishing Group, 1999.

4. Videos or VHS Formats (Additional Information)

The Brain: Our Universe Within
Discovery Channel, Discovery Communications, Inc.: Bethesda, MD, 1994.

The Secret Life of the Brain
PBS Series, David Grubin, Producer.

Afterword

STROKE RECOVERY IS a difficult ongoing task that necessitates constant work because it involves the center of your being—your brain. Finding my being and a gainful level of ability in my community and society is not easy. Moving from being a stroke patient to being an individual person again takes time, patience, determination, faith, and support. Here are a few positive affirmative statements that give me joy and reinforcement as I continue on my stroke recovery journey. Perhaps you can add your own items to the list.

* I must be healing from a stroke when:
* I open my eyes in the morning and I'm in my own bed.
* I can read the newspaper and the articles make sense.
* I can walk without assistance.
* I can eat, listen to table conversation, and swallow without choking.
* I can remember what program I'm watching on television.
* I can remember frequently used telephone numbers, including my own.
* I can get in and out of the bathtub by myself.
* I don't require a nap directly after getting dressed.
* I remember past events while focusing on the present.
* I make plans for the future even if I have to write them down.
* I keep a daily calendar just as I did before the stroke.
* I am oriented to the month, date, year, and day of the week most of the time.

* I don't know what it would be like living without thalamic (central) pain.
* I pay creditors on time and keep accurate financial records.
* I use a calculator and computer to assist in mathematic calculations.
* I can read an entire novel or story and comprehend, at least, the subject matter.
* I look forward to the future.
* I can follow a recipe and create a meal.
* I can crack an egg with one hand without getting eggshell into the dish.
* I can tie my shoes.
* I realize that naps are a great way to revitalize my brain.
* I think before I act.
* I think before I speak.
* I ask for assistance when needed.
* I understand emotional lability and try to avoid stressors or triggers like getting overtired.
* I understand the nuances of language enough to interpret facial expressions and tone.
* I understand a joke, pun, or humorous story.
* I laugh when things strike me as funny.
* I'm working on doing two things at the same time like thinking and smiling.
* I can simultaneously carry a plastic cup in my affected hand and walk a short distance.
* I can open a jar using a manual can opener.
* I take responsibility for my actions.
* I remember to feel water temperature with my unaffected hand.
* I remember to remove hot items from the stove or oven with my unaffected gloved hand.
* I consult with others before taking action on a major issue.
* I like myself and understand that, although the stroke was unfortunate, I am fortunate to be alive.
* I remember that perfection can only be achieved by the Almighty.

Some stroke experts say that there will never be a cure for stroke because stroke is not a disease, but a condition that is caused by other factors. Sadly, this may be true. However, we can fight for research that will provide for the early diagnosis of stroke in order to prevent permanent brain injury. As a stroke hero and advocate, I am keenly interested in stroke research. I believe that with the advance of medical technology, we are on the cusp of developing new techniques for the immediate diagnosis of stroke by emergency medical technicians (EMTs) and medical personnel in the field prior to reaching the hospital. Today, however, we must rely on educational efforts that reach out to everyone to teach them the warning signs of stroke. We, as a society, must fund research to develop medicines and support medical technology for faster diagnosis and treatment. With these advances in place, rapid diagnosis will be more readily available. Expedient diagnosis may translate into shorter recovery periods and soaring improvements in long-term disabilities. It is up to us. The future of stroke treatment depends on our global effort.

Men and women, boys and girls, all ages and abilities have been stricken with stroke—politicians to poultry farmers, celebrities to clerics, writers to welders, CEOs to chefs, movie directors to moguls, and everyone in between. Together, we have power. Together we can assist each other. We can team with corporations that have the technology we need to refine and assist us with home rehabilitation. Heroes of stroke helping heroes of stroke.

About the Author

CLEO HUTTON, *Stroke Hero, Author, Licensed Practical Nurse, Speaker, Advocate*

Cleo is a stroke hero/survivor, author/writer, professional speaker, Licensed Practical Nurse, educator, and advocate for stroke awareness and recovery. She is coauthor with Louis R. Caplan, MD, of *Striking Back at Stroke: A Doctor-Patient Journal* (Dana Press, 2003).

Hutton presents lectures around the world on the topic of stroke awareness and recovery. In February 2004, she was guest lecturer at the Department of Biochemistry, of the University of Coimbra, Portugal.

Cleo is a compassionate speaker who uses her heart, humor, and experience to deliver a message of hope and healing. She is a survivor of two strokes that initially rendered her without the ability to move or speak. After 12 years of what she calls "continuous rehab through everyday living," she is now able to communicate a message of hope and celebration. In so doing, Cleo breaks paradigms rooted in myths and misconceptions concerning stroke.

At the age of 43, Hutton had two right-side ischemic strokes, followed by heart surgery to repair a congenital heart defect. After formal rehabilitation, Hutton returned to college and graduated, at the young age of 50, with a Bachelor of Arts from the University of Minnesota. Through sheer determination and perseverance to regain control of her life, she attained Dean's List status and graduated with honors.

She has published articles in the American Stroke Association's

Stroke Connection and the National Stroke Association's *Stroke Smart* magazines. Cleo contributes a monthly article to The Stroke Network e-zine at www.StrokeNetwork.org and contributed the article "The Story of a Stroke Survivor," published in April 2001, on www.THRIVEnet.com, the Web site of Al Siebert, PhD. She wrote and published with www.StickYourNeckOut.com a humorous article, "Slipping the Ice Fantastic." Cleo is a member of the American Society for Training and Development and a member of Lake Superior Writer's group.

Hutton has presented at stroke survivor and caregiver conferences co-sponsored by the American Heart Association/American Stroke Association affiliates in Florida, Puerto Rico, Minnesota, Iowa, North Dakota, South Dakota, Washington, D.C., and elsewhere. In September 2003, Cleo Hutton received the Marion Rasmussen Award "for her dedication in educating others about stroke," presented by the Life After Stroke Committee in Minneapolis, Minnesota.

Cleo's campaign to spread the word about stroke and stroke rehabilitation has been carried on over 40 national radio shows and several television broadcasts, including CNN Health. Cleo Hutton is featured in *Prevention Magazine's* October 2003 issue, "It Could Happen to You" and *Cerebrum Magazine's* (Dana Press) October 2003 edition.

Cleo's mission is to foster independence for people living with stroke and to promote healing through a positive outlook.

Hutton is the mother of three adult children and a grandmother. She lives independently in northern Minnesota with her orange tabby cat, Buddy.

You may reach Cleo by e-mail at CleoHutton@aol.com.

Cleo Hutton is a pseudonym.

Index

NOTE: Boldface numbers indicate illustrations.

ischemic stroke, x

J

jar/can openers, 23, **24**
jewelry, 24
jokes. *See* humor and healing

K

kitchens, accessible changes to, 12, 23
knife, rocker type, 23, **23**
Knowledge and kindness in healing and building self-esteem, 37

L

large-print books and reading materials, 5-7
laughing inappropriately, 7-9
laundry, 54-56
    hanging clothes, 96
lawn care, 63
letters, writing and mailing, 89
love, 101-103
low-density lipoproteins (LDL) , xiii, xvi-xvii

M

making the bed, 58-59
MapQuest, 80
marriage and intimacy, 101-103
massage, 90
mattresses, 14
Meals on Wheels, 41
mealtimes, 47-49
medical care after stroke, xiii, xv, 123
medical conditions affecting stroke recovery, xiii-xiv
medical insurance coverage, 39-40
Medicare and Medicaid, 40
medications, 15-18, 85-86
    adverse interactions in, 15
    aspirin therapy and, 16-17
    bottle caps and, opening, 16
    contraindications to, 15
    diabetic, 18
    over the counter, 15
    prescription costs and, 38

shoulder, frozen, 90
shower chair, **20**, 20
showers and tubs, 11, 19-22
sickle-cell anemia, xiv, xvi
skin care
   deodorants and, 21-22
   moisturizers for, 21
sleep, 10
smoking, xvii
snow removal, 63-64
Social Security Disability Income (SSDI) benefits, 40-41
special equipment, 13-15
speech and language problems, xi, xviii-xx, 2-5
   family support in, 107-108
   idioms, clichés, and literal interpretation in, 5
   inappropriate speech in, 4-5
   overly talkative, 4-5
   understanding others, 3
   voice recognition software and, 92-93
stairs, 54-55
state assistance programs, 42
Strength in healing and building self-esteem, 35-36
Stroke Centers, xiii
Stroke Heroes, xviii
support groups, xviii
sweeping floors,, 57
swivel cushion for transfers, 26, 26

T

tape recorders, in reading comprehension, 6-7
TED stockings, 24-25, 28
teeth. *See* dental care
Telephone Equipment Distribution (TED) Program, 69
telephone skills, 69-71
television viewing, 91-92
THRIVEnet.com, 126
thromboembolism stockings (TEDs), 24-25, 28
Time in healing and building self-esteem, 36
tissue plasminogen activator (TPA), xiii
tobacco use, xvii
toenail care, 22, 30-31
toilet tissue, 96